RELEASE YOUR REGAIN

*Ignite Your Inner Power to Change
Your Body and Your Life*

Kristin Lloyd, MS, LPC/LMHC

Release Your Regain

DEDICATION

I'd like to dedicate this book to all those who have taken a chance on themselves. As bariatric patients, we've all gone through this surgery with the hopes it would be the final step on our road to weight loss. For many, it has been. For others, weight regain has been the hardest thing they have encountered. I want to acknowledge you for your strength and bravery on this journey back to yourself. You are fighting the fight each and every day. I see you, I believe in you, and I'm honored to be a guiding light on your journey to success.

CONTENTS

INTRODUCTION

Regain. It's the topic of blog articles, Facebook group topics, Twitter, and Instagram posts, and it's something that so many people freak out about.

Regain. What is it, and why does it happen?

Regain—that dreaded phrase no one ever wants to experience.

Regain. It's the thing bariatric patients fear most.

And, while there are biological, hormonal, and metabolic reasons, this book aims to cover the emotional, psychological, and behavioral reasons for weight regain after weight loss surgery.

If you believe that you've had a hormonal or metabolic reason for your weight regain, this book is not designed for you. As with anyone who experiences hormonal or metabolic changes, I would refer you back to the treating medical practitioner to conduct the appropriate medical testing.

For this book and its guidance, however, we will discuss the emotional, psychological, and behavioral reasons that can cause weight regain and ways to reverse it.

The shame that is experienced as a result of weight regain will also be covered. While many believe they have missed a window of opportunity, I'm here to share that you can release your regain at any time or stage of your journey. It just takes a recommitment to yourself and this bariatric journey. Through the foundational practices in this book, we'll take you through a series of steps and offer tools, strategies, and guidance to help you release your regained weight for good. If, at any time, you've lost your way, just come back to the beginning and start again. You can do it, you just need someone to help you along the way, and that is the aim of this book.

Now, let's get started!

CHAPTER 1

Re-Group and Get Ready

First, get real and honest with yourself about what you've been doing that has caused the regain.

It's time to be truthful with yourself about your journey so far. How and why regain happens is what we need to get clear on right now.

While people experience weight regain for many reasons, the most important one is how that happened for you.

When you practice awareness of what happened, you'll be able to prevent it from happening again.

In various talks I've given over the years and in all the research I've read, the majority of regain comes from poor lifestyle choices and a lack of behavior modification after surgery. The reason this happens is due to a lack of emotional support in the post-operative process, not enough discussions about behavior modification, and little education about the impact that lifestyle change will make in your weight loss journey long-term. Also, in the pre-op phase, everyone is eager to "just get the surgery already," not realizing what a tough and arduous journey it can be if unprepared.

Other issues could be contributing to your weight regain, such as hormone changes, autoimmune disorders, stress, and a lack of sleep. Still, the primary offender of regain is not making a permanent behavioral lifestyle change after surgery.

This book is not designed to shame or blame anyone. Instead, it's to guide and educate you on the war that is going on within you and around you every day. And, as I said in the introduction, this book focuses on the psychological, mental, emotional, and behavioral reasons for weight regain. If you feel your regain is due to a hormonal, biochemical, or is medical in nature, it is crucial you work with a medical practitioner to determine the root cause of the issue.

WHAT IS RESPONSIBLE FOR THE REGAIN

While a thousand reasons may have caused weight regain, the purpose here is to prepare and ready you for getting back on track. We hear that phrase a lot—back on track—and I'm sure it has a different connotation for everyone.

For some, it may mean being honest with yourself.

For some, it may mean sticking with a specific plan for longer than a few days.

For some, it may mean structure.

For some, it may mean overcoming emotional eating.

And, for others, it may be about what you're feeding your mind and your body.

The definition of the term *back on track* may change based on what it means to you.

To begin, I highly suggest that you come up with your own definition of *back on track* so you can see it clearly. Grab a sheet of paper, or maybe get a blank journal you can use while reading this book to help you process all that you are learning. Whatever you choose, for this activity, write down what you believe the term *back on track* means for you.

This is important because if it means deprivation or putting yourself on a diet, then let's work on changing that right now. Deprivation is linked to the "diet mentality," which is cyclical and typically and unfortunately ends in failure. Over and over, the cycle takes you through gaining, then dieting—maybe losing a bit—then going off the diet, and then feeling awful about yourself.

Is this how you want to live your life?

Ridding yourself of the diet mentality is one of the goals we will work toward in this book. Shifting your mindset from "diet" to "living healthy" is where we want you to be. This creates a balance and allows you to live more freely instead of restrictively. If you are in the "diet mentality," you likely have a belief system linked to how you eat and what you believe about food. Many diets are time-limited, and as a result, you believe you only must be on it for a while. The problem with this limited thinking is that you may go off the diet, resume old behaviors of overeating or using food to cope. Then you end up right back where you started. This cycle is why many diets do not work. Focusing on *lifestyle change* helps you integrate foods you desire and break the cycle of the diet mentality and deprivation.

REFLECTION QUESTIONS

Take out your notebook or paper and grab a pen. Reflect on the following questions and look at how your thinking about food may be impacting what you eat and how you eat. Several lists of reflection questions are included throughout the book, answer a few questions, or all of them. Think of them as journaling prompts, record the answers on your phone, or talk them over with an accountability buddy. Then reflect on what your answers say about your current relationship with food.

First, take a more in-depth look at your mindset around food and eating behaviors:

1. What do you think, or how do you feel about diets?
2. Do you hide food or impulsively choose foods that are higher in fat, sugar, or salt when you are struggling emotionally?
3. Do you eat "on the go" a lot? Do you eat in the car or standing up?
4. What do you think, or how do you feel about your favorite foods? Do they bring you shame after you eat them?
5. What is your definition of "healthy eating habits"?
6. What would it look like and feel like to eat healthily? Would you feel good about yourself? Or would you act out with foods you've deemed forbidden?

YOUR MINDSET ABOUT FOOD

Digging deeper into your understanding of how you see food and what you think about food, makes a big difference in how you interact with it. We each have our meanings for different phrases, and all of us have a specific engrained belief system that shapes the way we think about the foods we eat, the things we do, and the things we don't do. We have an interpretation or understanding of what is "good food" and what is "bad food."

A nutritionist taught me long ago that there is no such thing as "bad food" or "good food." Instead, I learned that there are foods to eat more often, foods to eat in moderation, and foods to eat sparingly.

This helped me to adjust my mindset about what foods might impact my body differently. Foods higher in sugar, for example, would be on my "sparingly" list because they might cause dumping, lethargy, or cravings. Foods higher in protein, for example, would likely fit the profile to be eaten more plentifully based on my post-bariatric lifestyle plan and ASMBS (American Society of Metabolic and Bariatric Surgery) nutritional guidelines. These high-protein foods are also helpful in maintaining muscle mass and keeping you fuller longer. The same would be true of fresh vegetables, which provide fiber and essential nutrients for your body's needs.

Research also suggests that those who change their plan to include healthy proteins along with vegetables, fruits, and complex low-glycemic carbohydrates are the most successful long-term.

This isn't about demonizing foods. Instead, it is about focusing on nutrient-rich foods while recognizing the impact and adverse effect foods higher in carbs and sugar may have on your body and brain. The foods you typically want more and more of are foods that are nutrient-poor but calorie-rich. These are foods that typically cause cravings. Looking at what foods you may be putting on a pedestal may also help you see a foundational issue regarding your relationship with food. Working on this issue will help heal your relationship with food and bring about awareness of how you may use food to cope with emotional stressors.

Recognizing what your patterns have been with food in the past, helps you regroup and get ready to alter these patterns. Awareness is vital when seeking to create a behavior change.

These OLD ways of interacting with food are not serving us or our new bodies and can only lead down that same path—to regain. Healing the old patterns and understanding the root causes will help create lasting behavior change.

A dear friend and colleague asked a question during training she gave; she asked, "Did we come all this way to have our bodies physically altered by surgery only to abuse them again with food?". I found this statement profound and alarming at the same time.

While some people might see this as harsh, I see it as a blunt question that sparks an awakening to the food issues that many continue to carry with them after surgery. Message boards and community groups on social media are filled with people asking the same questions: "When can I have Doritos again?" or, "When is it safe to have wine?" or, "How long do I have to wait until I can have bread?" and so on. While many are sincerely asking for advice, many don't even realize that going back to old habits can harm them, cause regain, and lead them right back to where they started. As I said before, we all have choices. We all have free will. I'm not the food police, and I don't plan on starting to be the food police anytime soon. Yet, this attitude is an important thing to examine when looking at the behavioral aspects of weight regain. When many are looking for a food-fix, not even a few weeks out of surgery, it can be seen as a cry for help or a yearning for something much more profound.

The emotional turmoil that many people battle is covered up by food, and, for many individuals, food is that coping mechanism. The thing is, they may not even see it.

For those having surgery in the United States, a pre-operative psychological evaluation is required to meet insurance requirements. In other places, it may not be a standard of care. Even so, many are approved for bariatric surgery and continue to struggle with food issues post-operatively because few places talk about the emotional struggles with food and how to adapt one's coping mechanism following this life-altering surgery. This oversight is why I believe it is essential to address this topic here. Many people only see what is needed to pass their pre-operative psychological exam and focus on getting the surgery as the final answer. You likely already know that the surgery is only a tool, and you must know how to use the tool. It isn't any different from how to wield a hammer. If you don't know how to use it, you could end up breaking a window.

The foundation for post-op care must go beyond what you need to eat in the first 8-10 weeks. You also need to know how to manage your emotions, how to handle other life challenges, and what to do when you see yourself going back to old behaviors. Sadly, not many post-op support groups cover this.

Post-op issues are life skills issues and largely emotional regulation issues. I've seen it over and over again. Many do great until they hit a bump in the road of life, and then boom, they get off track. They had the best of intentions to stay on track, but there wasn't a contingency plan. There wasn't a behavior plan to set them up—to set you up—for success, was there? This plan is what I want to share with you as part of this book.

What foods do you turn to when you've had a long day? What are the foods you turn to for comfort that you seek when bored, angry, lonely, or tired? It's time to get clear with yourself and not sugarcoat (no-pun intended) the response here. When people are hurting, they may turn back to food. When people are obese, struggling to move, struggling to live, and when they have tried absolutely everything, they seek surgery as a way to help them lose weight. Weight loss surgery can be an amazing blessing. Yet, when people haven't dealt with their food issues after surgery, they can go right back to the beginning and seek food for comfort. My goal is to help people rewire their brains and change their behaviors to do something else rather than reaching for food. It can be done.

When I had my surgery, my surgeon, who was a sleeve patient himself, gave me some sage advice. The day before my surgery, he told me, "You will reach a point in time that you will be able to get in excess of 3,000 calories per day if you want to, but you won't want to, it will just happen. Believe me, you'll need to stay vigilant and pay attention to what you're eating. Focus on meals, not snacks. Beware of grazing behaviors. Get your water in and be consistently mindful of what you're eating. If you do that and you change your behaviors, you'll be fine."

This advice has stayed with me ever since. This straight talk frightened me, but it also kept me focused on what I'm doing to nourish my body. I want to pass this advice on to you as well. The old habits that you've held on to, for whatever reason, will not help you open new doors or new ways, and they won't get you to where you want to be.

About four weeks after surgery, I had a wake-up call. I was still on soft foods at the time. I craved a cheeseburger and wanted one so bad that I figured out a way to make it happen. On my approved foods list was pate. Pate was ground meat, or so I thought. I rationalized what it was and decided that I could put some cooked ground beef in a blender with some cheese, in order to make homemade pate. I even had to add water so it would get mixed up. Believe me, it was gross looking in the blender, but I just had to have it. After I ate a few small spoonfuls of the mixture I had concocted, I experienced such bad stomach pain that I was laid up on the couch for a few hours, doubled over in pain. I didn't hurt my sleeve, thank goodness, but I did recognize that I had a problem, and cheeseburgers—in any form—were not the solution. Even after this episode, I challenged my pouch a few times more. Each time, my pouch (or sleeve) would respond by making saliva bubble-up in my mouth, letting me know that I would have to throw up soon. My husband always called my pouch "the Civic." He had named it this because he said that my weight loss surgery cost as much as a Honda Civic. It was a reminder that not only had I altered my body, but I had done so in an extreme way so that I could be healthy. My behaviors, however, were not healthy.

This wake-up call was the beginning of my own journey to get healthy, not only physically, but also mentally and emotionally. It wasn't easy, and it was a long road that started with honesty and coming to terms with emotions that I didn't want to face. My own battles with food led me to some harsh realities about how I used food to cope. And, as I shared above, most people have to go through a pre-operative psychological evaluation. I went through this same evaluation with a psychological professional, but it didn't guarantee my success or my readiness to deal with my own emotional hang-ups with food. It was through the journey after having surgery that I had to walk the walk, day after day, practicing my awareness with food and recognizing my behavioral patterns with food. Based on my own personal journey and working with thousands of other bariatric patients, I know that this isn't just about the surgery and the food. It's also about emotions and mindset, and it is from this vantage point that I teach.

The shame that I experienced after the cheeseburger blender incident impacted me. I felt awful about myself. Although no one else knew other than my immediate family, the self-talk inside my head had resurrected my inner hateful, mean girl like no other. Shame leads us to eat more, not less. This negative voice made me want to eat more, not less. Her daily barrage of hate, judgment, criticism, and putdowns made me want to eat more, not less. So, I had to do something about that shame if I was going to get healthy. I had to break free from the voice. I had to get help.

Once again, however, my own inner work was the only way to come to terms with that inner mean girl and the shame so that I wouldn't repeatedly turn to food. I had to be ready to do the work. That is the key point here, and the whole point of this chapter. It's about *readiness*. Some people aren't ready to do the work or to look deep inside themselves. The point here is not to shame anyone or point fingers but to compassionately say that things won't get better until you get yourself ready. Trying to do the work and not being ready only leads to more pain, more stress, and more shame. If you're not ready, we'll talk more about getting ready and what that looks like. Each and every person has their own journey to readiness. Being ready for change is a step in and of itself.

After my own harsh realization that I had some work to do, I started to write things down about what was popping up in my head. I started to pay attention to the voice of my inner mean girl. I also started journaling to talk to myself in a more loving, supportive, and compassionate way. I would write all the hateful things this mean girl would say, and then I would challenge them. Recording this conversation in my head is how I started to journal. I didn't start by having fancy prompts. I just wrote the dialogue between the mean girl and my other inner voice, whom I've named "the encourager."

Let's also be clear here; I know that not everyone will journal out their emotions or feelings. I've met many people who are resistant to it, and I'm aware of that. For those, I highly suggest that you speak into a voice recorder so that you can get those thoughts outside of your head. This way, you can reflect on what your own inner mean voice says so you can combat the violent vitriol that your negative cyclical self-talk regularly spews. You can also call it out, reframe it, and shift it in a healthy, loving, and productive way. Being the truth-teller and truth-seeker is possible only when you see what's on the table. When the negative voices stay inside your head, you may not be able to call it out or shift it.

I tell my clients regularly; your inner voice has no filter. That mean girl says things you would NEVER say to your best friend or loved one because you have a socialized filter that acknowledges it as unacceptable. You wouldn't tell your best friend that she is an ugly fat pig. You wouldn't tell your child that he or she is a loser who will never succeed. Yet, we say these things to ourselves. We regularly criticize, shame, and judge ourselves, with our own inner voice.

There's no way to filter through these negative thoughts when you fully believe them. One of my mentors used to say, "Don't believe everything you think.", this is so true! How often do you believe what that negative voice says like it's the gospel? When you take these negative thoughts and put them down on paper or say them out loud in a voice recorder and then listen to them back, you can combat them. You can reality check them. You can say, "Wait a minute, this is BS!" Only when you can filter through them, can you recognize that your self-talk is likely perceived through a negative or fearful lens. When you're able to look at these thoughts (either on paper or in voice form), you can consciously challenge them, and everything changes. You can change your thoughts once you're aware of them. You can change your thoughts, and you can choose new ones. You can choose thoughts that are encouraging, loving, kind, and compassionate.

Journaling became part of my own therapeutic process. It helped me get out of my head so that I could separate the "mean girl" from the girl who so badly wanted to change her life for the better.

This separation was the beginning of a healing experience for me, and it led to continued weight loss followed by maintenance. Had I not worked on healing, I know that I would have been a regain statistic, and I didn't want to go there. This knowledge is why I have so much compassion and love for those who have experienced weight regain. I know pain and hurt are being covered up by food. This knowledge is why I am writing this today, so that I can help you change your own mindset around food and to heal your own issues with food, for good.

When Molly, 56, came to work with me, she had struggled with her own inner mean girl. After experiencing a regain of 32 pounds at four years post-op, she was frightened she would "gain it all back." She admitted she used food to soothe when she had a rough day at work, or when she felt she "deserved" a break from the hardships she experienced in her day-to-day life. The truth was, she was abusing food to soothe or to avoid dealing with her emotions. Additionally, her own inner mean girl was loud, and man, was her negative voice vile! We worked through her triggers, urges, and the emotions that surfaced when she struggled the most. This helped her to get a hold on the inner mean girl and to talk to herself differently. However, before our work together, she didn't even realize she was berating herself on a regular basis. She hadn't realized how hard she was on herself or the expectations she had of herself. It was through practicing awareness and changing her self-talk that she started to see when she would usually turn to food. Through her readiness for change, she was able to tackle the challenges that the inner mean girl voice presented. People often think that dealing with food is first. However, food can often be a symptom of a deeper issue. Starting with "what you're eating" may not necessarily be the first step. The "what" you eat can be a symptom of "why" you eat. The "why" (you eat) may be more important to tackle at first so that you can properly address the "'what."

Emily, 42, came to me during a period when she had experienced weight regain of 47 pounds. She recalled the shame and anger at herself for letting her emotional eating get out of control. We briefly discussed her patterns with food. She shared her food intake and shared that she had gone back to eating protein bars and protein shakes in an attempt to get control of her behaviors. While this wasn't immediately alarming, as she continued talking about it, it became clear that she prioritized these processed foods over nutrient-rich foods. She also said they helped her avoid other challenging foods, which caused her to overeat.

While the processed foods did not create her regain, they weren't helping her to lose the weight either. She also mentioned that they sometimes added to her cravings, which caused her to eat more on occasion.

Emily's experience is why it is so important to look at the nutritional content of the foods you are eating and how processed they may be. Some chemicals can increase cravings. Learning to meal prep, cook, and create meals from REAL food is part of the post-operative process for a lifestyle change. This ensures you know what is in your food, so you have greater control over what you eat.

Agnes, 68, also wanted to change her relationship with food. She had regained 32 pounds as an 8-year post-operative RNY patient when she contacted me. She recognized she went back to seeking convenience foods, mainly fast-food and pizza. She would particularly eat when she would have a stressful day and reward herself with food. Agnes was still working and shared that she expected to work at least a few more years before retiring. She wanted to be healthy and struggled with managing her food choices. Her exhaustion at the end of each day left little time for meal prep, and she hadn't integrated new patterns of lifestyle change into the daily routine. This impacted her food choices, and, since she was not aware of her "food as reward" pattern, she continued to state that something was wrong with her.

In fact, there was and is nothing wrong with Agnes. She was just committed to a certain pattern of behaviors that were not serving her, her body, or her long-term goals. In our work together, we created a plan to help her change her mindset and her behaviors around food. She still was able to make her own pizza at home on occasion, without the guilt when it met the guidelines of her food plan. The food she made at home was easy to pull together, and she learned how to manage her time and her priorities, as well as how to shift the focus away from food as a reward. She also learned how to eat when she was out so she could stay on plan when out with friends. She now saw food as nourishment and was able to not only make better choices with food, but she was also able to feel good about what she was eating. She was less fatigued and more in control of her eating behaviors.

Looking at these examples of others who have struggled with food, it becomes clear that creating a new relationship with food begins, in the mind. We can know "what" to eat, but if we aren't getting to the core of "why" we eat, it does not matter how many awesome recipes you have in your possession. When you can take food off the pedestal and recognize the limiting beliefs that you carry around yourself, around food, and around your habits and behaviors, you are then able to create new routines, new beliefs, and new patterns of behavior that lead you to the life and body you desire.

BEING READY FOR CHANGE

Prior to recommitment, you also need to know where you stand. Being ready is a process. It's not something you flip the switch on, although we all wish we could.

The Transtheoretical Model of Behavior Change (TTM) is the leading model of health behavior change. TTM was developed in the 1970s by Dr. James Prochaska and his colleagues at the University of Rhode Island and has been the topic of many studies. It is an integrative theory of therapy that evaluates an individual's readiness to act upon a new healthier behavior. It is comprised of "stages of change" in which individuals move through as a process of growth in health behavior. It is used in health theory, addiction research, and other health-related practices.

The stages are classified as follows:

Precontemplation – (not ready for a change) In this stage, individuals are in denial or completely unaware that their behavior is problematic. They are not ready to change and have no plans to change in the foreseeable future.

Contemplation – (getting ready for a change) Individuals have an awareness that their behavior is problematic. In this stage, they begin to look more closely at the path they are on, along with the risks and rewards of change.

Preparation – (ready for a change) In this stage, individuals intend to make changes and take action soon, within the immediate future. They may also begin to take small steps toward a healthy behavior change.

Action – In this stage, individuals have begun to make specific behavior modifications, changing habits, reducing problem behaviors, and working on practicing new healthy behaviors.

Maintenance – In this stage, individuals have sustained action for a minimum of six months and are consistently working to prevent relapse.

Termination – In this stage, individuals have zero temptation to go back to their old (unhealthy) behaviors, and they are certain they will not return to this previous method of coping.

(Relapse) – This is not an official stage of behavior change; however, it is regarded in the literature as important to discuss, as relapse can happen in any stage where individuals return to an earlier stage of change (typically moving them from maintenance to action).

Getting you acquainted with this model of behavior change is essential, as you may need to get clear on where you stand. If you are not ready for change, beating yourself up over and over for not taking action is not going to do any good. If you are not ready for change, then instead of blaming or shaming yourself, look deeper at what you can do to get ready for change.

Similarly, if you are in the action phase, but keep relapsing, it is important to recognize what is causing relapse so that you can gain clarity, make changes, and move forward.

This knowledge will help you regroup and get ready to release weight regain and help you stay on track for good. When you know that you may have a propensity for relapse, you might pay closer attention to your triggers and behaviors. Knowing these stages of change also helps you recognize that you are not failing but, instead, may need more preparation in your readiness for change.

PROCESSED FOODS, FOOD AS STIMULUS, &
THE FAST FOOD INDUSTRY

You're likely programmed to seek out the sugary, fatty, and salty foods that are reinforced by the pleasure centers of your brain. You're likely not sure how to self-soothe when bad things happen in your life, and so you go back to old coping mechanisms—one of those being food.

You're likely also programmed to eat what is fast and easy, which may be loaded with a lot of processed chemicals. When you eat a lot of these foods, your brain then craves foods with significant processed chemicals. Thus, the cycle repeats itself over and over.

For a moment, humor me here. Let's take a quick look at foods, stimulus, and advertising. Have you noticed what foods are being advertised? Are they the foods that are healthy? Or are they the foods that lead to cravings? The fast-food and convenience food industries are multi-billion-dollar industries—just like the DIET industry. In my last book, *Bariatric Mindset Success: Live Your Best Life and Keep the Weight Off, After Weight Loss Surgery*, I talked about the diet industry and their desire to sell you quick fixes, which end up taking your money and leaving you feeling like a failure. The newest "thing," whether it is a pill, product, device, or gadget, have you believing that this *ONE thing* will be your final savior. The latest and greatest thing will save you from obesity and appeals to your desperation to lose weight. So, you buy it. You buy it with your heart filled with hope that you'll lose the weight. The problem is that NONE of those gadgets, gizmos, or pills show you how to STICK with something. Before you know it, you end up back to your old routine, not using the gizmo or gadget, and you end up feeling like a failure again. The problem is not the product itself; it's about your behavior change. The mindset shift within you is what you need in order to USE the product long-term, but no one tells you that. The bottle of pills, product, device, gizmo, or gadget, ends up on a shelf in the garage or tucked away into a closet. Behavior change is key, and that's NOT what sells, so they continue to sell you what you will buy: products, pills, and devices.

What you're really buying, though, is HOPE. A hope that things will change. A hope that things will be different this time. The device, pill, or product won't change you—only YOU can change you. Only YOU have the power to change you.

The fast-food industry also gets you in this way. They have cornered the market on fast, quick, and easy. They know what you need and why you need it, and they make it specifically for you. They offer "healthy" options on the menu, yet there are more unhealthy options than healthy ones. They know you need something fast and quick. This leads you to rely on willpower to make a healthy choice. When you are already running late, hungry, anxious, tired, and/or running low on funds, you can't rely on willpower. Studies show that when you're in a psychologically vulnerable state, you cannot rely on willpower. The fast-food industry counts on this, too. Many of the healthy options are also more expensive, leading consumers to choose an unhealthy and cheaper option.

It has been estimated that fast-food companies spent over $4 billion dollars on advertising in 2019 alone. A 2012 study showed that the fast-food industry marketed their most unhealthy products specifically to children and teens as their key audience despite having "healthy options" on the menu. According to the Yale University Rudd Center for Food Policy & Obesity, fast-food companies spent approximately $4.6 billion on advertising in 2012 (Orciari, 2018).

Within these advertisements, social leaders, such as stars, athletes, actors, and famous individuals, are used to insert "authority" that suggests not only is the food good but also it must be acceptable to eat. Even the Olympic games are sponsored by fast-food companies. The athletes get endorsements, and everybody is happy, right? These actors and athletes are getting paid millions of dollars to eat burgers, tacos, pizza, fries, and soda on TV to tickle your taste buds and to get you to open your wallet. Fast-food companies contribute to noble causes, which also plays on your heartstrings. They must be good because they are sponsoring the Special Olympics and helping kids to read, right? Their key to your wallet is creative; they show you athletes and actors who must be fit in order to excel, which conflicts with the truth. These athletes are seen eating this junkie food, yet in order to keep their healthy physiques and maintain their athletic abilities, they are most definitely NOT eating these types of foods on the regular. Kind of a conundrum, right?

The ads target you, the consumer. They use famous people whom you look up to and social capital to get you to buy into their product. Absolutely genius, right?

These foods may be fast, easy, and cheap, but over time, it's expensive for your health. The food you pay for on the dollar menu, or two-for-five-dollar menu, for example, will end up costing you thousands if not hundreds of thousands of dollars in health care costs over time. The food you eat is directly related to your body's health. High blood pressure, high cholesterol, diabetes, and obesity have all been linked to an overabundance of calories and a lack of nutrition. Most obese patients are malnourished. It's not about the weight. It's about the nutrition they are getting. Many convenience foods and fast foods are low in nutrition and high in calories. See the issue?

Most of the foods you eat from these fast-food places may taste good, but that's because they add chemicals and process the food to make sure you come back for more. These foods are considered 'highly palatable foods,' which means that they target your taste receptors, creating food memories to ensure you come back for more. These highly palatable foods are typically higher in sugar, fat, and salt (the trifecta), which Dr. David Kessler talks about in his book *The End of Overeating*.

Americans are particularly attached to fast food as part of a mainstream diet, which is just one way our country has been led into an obesity crisis, all while creating a robust income for the fast-food industry. Fast-food companies also target individuals with a lower socioeconomic status—people who live in poorer neighborhoods—consequently driving up obesity in those areas.

The fast-food industry has you right where they want you. In their eyes, you need them. They satisfy your cravings, their prices are right, and that's why they are on the television consistently advertising with neurolinguistic programming, a marketing tool they use to suggest you have a desire for your food, even when you may not be hungry. When you see a fast-food commercial at 10 p.m. at night, you have that urge to place an order right away via your phone or computer and have one of the local companies deliver. They've made it so easy for you to purchase from them. The advertising cost is a drop in the bucket compared to what Americans spend on average to eat fast food.

Just out of curiosity, have you ever seen a broccoli or carrot campaign? Have you ever noticed a television advertisement making blueberries or strawberries look sexy? I bet you haven't, and I doubt you ever will.

I distinctly remember an ad a few years back that caught my attention. It was a burger ad. There was a woman wearing a string bikini on the hood of a car, with her hair flowing in the wind, eating a double beef patty cheeseburger. The fast-food industry does everything they can to make their food look sexy and appealing. And, they are marketing to YOU.

Do these companies have your best interest at heart? Are they concerned about your health, or making more money? Are their marketing campaigns designed to help you get healthy and happy? Or are their campaigns designed to sell more fast food regardless of whether you are frustrated, angry, or obese?

Whose interests do they have in mind when they advertise? Ever notice that they always show thin people eating their foods, too? This is also an advertising trick to make the food seem acceptable. If they showed obese individuals in these ads, or if they showed you what would look like after 30 days of eating their food like in the documentary *Supersize Me*, they wouldn't make any money.

This is all about making more money at your expense. They do their best to create a 'cheaper' product so that you'll buy it, and they market primarily to those who struggle financially. Doesn't that sound twisted? They do that to ensure they have you roped in. They make a product that is highly palatable, filled with sugar, salt, and fat to make sure you come back for more, all while keeping it within your budget. It sounds like a great product, right? Err... Or is it?? Maybe it tastes good. Or, maybe it's great until you have to see the doctor and then you get hit with a $3,568 medical bill for the MRI, CT scan, blood work, and, ohh yes, the blood pressure and cholesterol meds that you'll be taking. This happens all while the doctor tells you to "watch your diet."

Sound familiar?

These ads come on during prime-time television, they come on late at night, and they are looking for you. They come on when they expect you're watching, and they have you right where they want you. They are programming you to crave their foods, and they are programming your mind to desire what they are selling.

Here's another point to keep in mind. Your "diet" as they call it, is not ONLY what you eat, it's everything that you consume—what you watch on television, what you read, what you listen to, etc. So, as you work to shift your mindset, be mindful of everything you are consuming, and ask yourself, is it worth it? Ask yourself, is this getting me where I want to go? Is this helping me achieve my goals? Or is this making it harder for me to achieve my goals because it's programming me to do what they want me to do? Think about it.

So, I've got to ask you, is eating cheap worth it? Is eating fast food worth it? Are you willing to exchange your health for something quick and easy?

Aren't you worth more than that? I firmly believe you are. And that's why I'm writing this to you because it's gone on for way too long. I don't know who you are personally, but I know you've picked up this book for a reason. My purpose is to help guide people back to themselves, and to put them back in the driver's seat of their lives. I've seen so many of my bariatric clients, friends, and colleagues struggle with food. This is why I've felt called to teach the mindset aspects of food. The food itself is just an entity. It's a symptom of a greater issue.

Advertising speaks to your mindset. It speaks to all the triggers inside your head. It speaks to your urges, your cravings, and your desires. These advertisements are sexy, and they romance the hell out of you, and BOOM, you buy-in.

But let me get real for a second, this isn't about calling out the food industry, although I think I've done a damn good job of doing that just now. We live in a society where we all have free will and can make our own choices. What I want to bring to light here is this: when you don't have control over your mind, there are entities that will persuade you to do what they want you to do, and it may not always be with your best interest or with your greatest health in mind. You *do* have a choice. You have a choice to do something differently. You have control over what you watch. You have control over what you allow into your mind and your body. You have the choice to live differently.

The focus of this book is to help you see that it's not just the food you choose to eat that is causing the regain, but also the excitement and stimulus that is created around food and the experience inside your brain. The advertising creates this fictionalized experience that is exciting and stimulating. It makes you go, "Ooooh ..." Prior to having bariatric surgery, I spent a lot of time watching the Food Network. It was food porn. They made it hot and sexy. I realized after surgery that I had the power to choose what I was watching and how it affected me, my mind, my taste buds, and my food desires. So, I changed the channel. I put my mind back in control. Truth be told, these days I spend a lot more time reading than I do watching television, and this is because I want to control what I am feeding my mind.

If you put yourself in a position where food becomes a central focus, it can be torture, especially if you are condemned for how you look and struggling with your desire, how you look, and how you feel. This starts when you are tantalized and tempted and then told by the diet industry, "nope, you can't have that." This creates deprivation, shame, guilt, and many other emotions. However, if you aren't constantly bombarded with food messages, you might not think about food all the time, either. We can't change the food industry. We can't change advertising. The only thing we can change, and have the power to change is ourselves.

This is why it's deeper than the food. It's about the messages and whom you allow to be in charge of your mind.

Grocery store aisles aren't any better, sadly. As I've shared before, processed foods can be quick and easy, but they may not be the best for your body. Additionally, there are many quick processed and convenience food products that have been designed specifically for the bariatric community. However, those "food products" may not be "foods" at all.

Many are just as processed as the junk food you find in the grocery store, and this shows in the body's ability to process them. If you don't believe me, try reading the ingredients on the package. This isn't about any one food product either; it's about educating you about what you are putting in your body.

These pre-packaged foods with ingredients you can't name, let alone pronounce, can also cause food triggers from your pre-op life or potentially lead you to eat more and more of these "snack" type processed foods. One of the biggest offenders found in many processed foods is maltodextrin. While it is generally marked as a safe ingredient, when people eat too many processed foods, their diet is likely to be lower in fiber and higher in sugar overall. Maltodextrin has an even higher glycemic index than table sugar (Schafer, A., Baker, L., & Gotter, A., 2017; Silva, 2018). Therefore, when people eat a lot of products packed with maltodextrin, they may experience a spike in blood sugar even if they are not eating sugary foods. Eating a plethora of foods with maltodextrin can lead to an increase in blood sugar and, over time, can be linked with diabetes. Maltodextrin, in large amounts, can also negatively impact gut bacteria, which is essential for overall health and immune function (Schafer, A., Baker, L., & Gotter, A., 2017; Silva, 2018).

When you eat more and more of these types of foods, you're obviously eating less and less of the natural foods that are packed with the necessary nutrients which your body needs. Overall, reading food labels is important, and knowing what is inside the foods we are eating is essential for health. Many of us expect the government to regulate food products and food ingredients, yet ultimately, we as consumers have an obligation to decide what to put in our bodies.

While I don't expect any of us to get rid of ALL these foods because they can be a supplement for many, my point here is to help you get better at living an 80/20 life. Living 100% clean is not the point here. Everyone needs supplementary foods and on the go choices. The more you create balance and practice awareness of what you're regularly eating, the easier it becomes to maintain your weight. Additionally, as a quick supplement in one's overall food plan, these can be foods that are part of the 20% of one's life. If a food plan includes 50% or more of these foods, an impact on weight and blood sugar would be expected, as well as possible contributions to other health issues. Individuals may not recognize these foods as a danger, nor understand what it is happening, especially after weight loss surgery. Discussing it here is intended to help you be more informed about food products, what is inside them, and how you can take control over your choices back. The more you know about what is in your food, the better choices you can make.

LIVING THE 80/20 LIFE

Prior to surgery, I led a 20/80 life. I ate 20 percent healthy food and 80 percent fast food, junk food, and/or processed food. This diet is the main reason I had to have surgery. I abused my body. I ate crap. I ate for taste and not for health. I fell into the trap of processed, pre-packaged, convenience, and fast foods. Pizza and Cheetos were my all-time top foods of choice. This is how I know what I know about lifestyle change and obesity. I've been there. I've done the research, and I've had to work on my own mindset to avoid going back there. I tried for many years to "diet" to lose weight. My weight loss would get capped at 50 pounds, and then the gain/loss cycle would begin again. I couldn't get passed that 50-pound mark. It was frustrating. This cycle is why I had weight loss surgery. I had so much more to lose, and my body would just stop at that initial 50 pounds, no matter how much energy I put into my dieting process. I worked out hard and strength trained. I was upsetting because I put so much into it, and the weight loss wasn't there. So, I would go back to old habits—eating junk and giving up. This book shows you how I've come to turn it all around. I've used weight loss surgery as a transformative process and as an opportunity to shift my mindset around food and eating.

What I do now is lead an 80/20 life, that is, 80 percent healthy whole foods filled with protein (beef, fish, chicken, pork, tofu, etc.), fresh fruits and vegetables, and a moderate amount of healthy complex carbohydrates (quinoa, flax, chia, legumes, oats, etc.). This helps my body stay nourished and within a healthy caloric range for a post-op bariatric patient.

What I am a proponent of is helping people create this 80/20 mindset in their own life so they can achieve the same. Also, while so many see this to be about food, it is really about the mindset around the food.

Whether it's processed foods or fast foods, no one is going to rid their diet of 100% of these foods, unless they are living toward the extreme. In our community, any extremes lead to more problems, not less. Any average individual, however, can adopt an 80/20 lifestyle, with 80% of their foods coming from whole, healthy sources, and less than 20%

coming from processed/convenience foods or fast foods. This creates a healthier balance and is sustainable.

Some people may believe they can't sustain this ratio. You know who you are—especially those who struggle with sugar, simple carbohydrates, and white flour. Again, I repeat, you know who you are. This goes back to the principle, "Know thyself." If you are one of these individuals who may grapple with or need to come to terms with your struggle with these foods, I strongly encourage meeting with an eating disorders therapist or a nutritionist who specializes in helping you with food elimination. Not everyone needs food elimination or requires abstinence from white flour and sugar. Yet, there are many who must live this way in order to avoid binging or experiencing other issues that represent behaviors consistent with an eating disorder. I have seen many people who need to release these foods for good, not only for their physical wellbeing but also for their own mental health. I don't believe in a one size fits all. It is all about achieving a balance in your life and in what works for you. It is all about knowing yourself, first and foremost. The purpose here is to guide you to a lifestyle that is livable for you, for the long-term. I've had so many clients who have told me of their struggles with simple sugars and white flour, which becomes a daily battle. Other people can have one bite and are fine. Knowing who you are and what impacts you is essential for releasing your regain and living this lifestyle long-term.

EMOTIONAL EATING

Emotional eating can be one of the major issues that lead to weight regain. Over time, using food to soothe complex emotional states leads to a behavioral pattern that one doesn't even recognize. Often, I'll have clients say, "I don't even know how that food ended up in my mouth." One minute they were in a meeting, and the next, they ended up with chips or chocolate in their mouth. This type of behavior is what I refer to as "autopilot eating." This is the behavioral pattern that is developed through the reward circuitry of the brain. In order to escape difficult feelings, people reach for a food that stimulates the reward center of their brain in order to feel better. The neurotransmitters released are typically dopamine, serotonin, and endorphins. Endorphins can also be released through physical activity. However, if someone has been programmed to get this from food, it is part of their inherent behavioral programming.

There was a time when I recognized that the food I was eating was hurting me. I knew I was harming myself, and I did it anyway. I didn't know how else to cope with the emotions.

And... at that time, I didn't even realize it was my emotions that were driving me to eat.

So, rather than feel, or deal, I ate. This was how I landed at over 400 pounds, to begin with! This is likely how you ended up where you were, to begin with too. The goal is NOT to go back there, and some people dealing with regain are already back there. So how do you get back on track?

You've got to deal with "the stuff."

I avoided dealing with the stuff—the issues, the feelings, the boundaries, the responsibility, the shame, the guilt... all of it... I AVOIDED.

It made me feel icky and yucky. Who wants to deal with their feelings??

After surgery that I realized I had an anxiety disorder. All that time as a pre-op, I thought I was "dealing" with things. As it turns out, I was coping with food. When the anxiety appeared, my brain was on the search for food. I wasn't physically hungry, either. I would find myself standing in front of the refrigerator, looking for something. I would stop myself recognizing that it was neither time to eat, nor was I physically hungry. I wanted "something" to take the edge off. I recognized I was an emotional eater.

One of the things I recognized after surgery was how deep the wounds went, and how often I'd used food to cope and to self-soothe.

I learned this lesson when I tried to return to old foods and became violently ill ... remember what I shared earlier??

My pouch said, "Oh, hell, no, we are not doing that anymore!"

As if my pouch could talk—HA—but it was loudly yelling into the toilet nonetheless ...

Dumping and getting sick doesn't happen for everyone, and I realized at that moment, getting sick after eating to self-soothe was a blessing, not a curse. I did not want to go backward. I did not want to fail my pouch. I had to do something different, and I had to work on myself. This was when the true mindset of work began.

Working through the feelings and uncovering, which made me feel uncomfortable was the beginning of it all. "Becoming comfortable with being uncomfortable" became a motto for a while as well. Many others still struggle with this piece, and I understand why. In psychology, we talk about pain vs. pleasure principle. Many seek out pleasure and avoid pain. Food is pleasurable, and so to avoid dealing with uncomfortable emotions, food can be an easy out. In this process, however, finding new alternative routes to cope is essential to avoid regaining the weight. Weight regain is also leads to a host of other emotions and, of course, other health issues.

Healing the emotions is one piece; dealing with the regain is another. Following a path to healthy eating and healing, one's relationship with food is significant in this process. When people return to problem foods, it is usually a symptom of a bigger issue, but not the core issue itself.

In my work with many individuals (mostly women), I realized that not everyone has the blessing of getting sick. Some people can eat whatever, whenever...

Some people return to soda. Some people return to slider foods, and they graze. Some people push the food down to fit more in...

Some people aren't aware that they are making themselves sicker by returning to old habits. And, some of them know it...

The point here is not to blame, shame, or guilt anyone into getting back on track—however, I often am asked, "WHAT CAN I DO?"

Well, while I'm always a proponent of going back to the basics ... before that, you MUST recommit to yourself AND ... recommit to the process of GIVING UP WHAT MAKES YOU SICK!

I have a LOT of compassion for struggling folks.

I really do.

But the answer is not in forcing a change if you're not ready...

Instead, you need to start the process of GETTING READY for the changes you desire to make.

When you say one thing and do another—you're clearly not ready to recommit. You may SAY you want it ... but your actions display that you're not actually ready.

So, instead of hating on yourself for not being ready and potentially repeating old behavior patterns, you MUST get ready to recommit.

The cycle of blame, shame, and guilt can be so strong that you may repeat negative cycles because you don't know how to cope.

So today, whether it's you or someone you know and love—I'm going to help you get ready.

In typical fashion, I'm going to give you some steps to prepare for the journey ahead ...

HOW DO YOU RECOMMIT?

Before recommitting yourself to yourself, your bariatric journey, your post-op bariatric life, and to your bariatric basics, you've got to address the following:

Acknowledge the patterns that continue to keep you stuck and/or sick

How important is it to you to STAY sick? Especially if your patterns are continuing to perpetuate the sickness.

How important it is for you to get WELL, including prioritizing your WELLNESS, and new LIFESTYLE choices.

This is how you begin stepping into RE-COMMITMENT.

Ask yourself: What is making me sick? What is keeping me stuck?

What are the habits, foods, coping mechanisms, behavioral responses, etc., that continually make you sick? This doesn't always necessarily mean the things that create physical sickness. Include the things, food, and behaviors that also lead to emotional sickness. What foods trigger you? What foods hold you emotionally hostage or make you feel guilty? What behaviors or coping mechanisms do you engage in that make you feel awful about yourself? What activities, coping mechanisms, or food push you backward instead of driving you forward?

WRITE THEM OUT. Make a list of the things that push you backward, that end up hurting you in the long run, that you reach for when you're stressed or struggling, and that lead you off track consistently.

Then, really look at this list.

Stare at it.

Get super real with yourself.

Add more commentary if it helps you see the patterns of behavior or the foods/habits/behaviors that are keeping you sick and stuck.

Ask yourself: What happens if nothing changes?

Play this story out in your journal. Where will you be in a year, five years, ten years, if absolutely NOTHING changes? If you continue using the habits, foods, coping mechanisms, and behaviors that continually make you sick, or return you to your pre-op self...

How would you feel?

What would life be like?

What would that mean for you?

Ask yourself: Why do I need it?

When it comes to specific foods, you likely have an automatic reaction, not a response. This leads you to repeat the same behaviors over and over again. Getting clear on why you need these foods or why you want them may help you come to terms with your behavioral patterns. Ask yourself why you need these things? What do they provide for you? What do they give you? How are they benefitting your life? What's the draw to these foods or behaviors? Are they exciting or stimulating? Do they numb you? Do they stop boredom for a few moments? Are they really that important? Are they more important than your goals?

Asking yourself some deeper questions helps you realize that you may be reacting to your environment or to conditional situations rather than making conscious choices. You likely feel a great draw to certain foods that pull you in, over and over again. The purpose here is to help you gain a deeper understanding of this draw so that you can change your behavior over time.

Ask yourself: How is this impacting my goals? How is this impacting whom I want to become?

This is a great reflection activity. When you get clear on whom you want to be, you can start to see how your day-to-day actions might be preventing you from getting there. If you are consistently hitting the drive-through on the way into work and then shaming yourself later in the day, how is that helping you change? Or is it just causing more pain?

It is essential to start asking yourself what you truly desire. What are your goals? Whom do you want to become beyond your weight loss journey? What would it be like to reach goal weight or close to it? What would it be like to be a smaller pant size? How would that feel? Whom do you want to become in all aspects of your life? What would that mean to you? How will achieving your weight loss goals change your life? What would you get to do once you have achieved your weight loss goals?

Answering these questions may help you gain additional clarity.

People in this process are often also afraid of reaching their goals and subconsciously sabotage their process. Often in my practice, I meet with individuals in this situation, and they engage in the same behaviors that keep them stuck to avoid other consequences. It may be that being smaller or thinner makes them feel physically unsafe, so they have avoided it even though a part of them wants it so badly. This is something to keep in mind, as well. Are you afraid of reaching your goals for one reason or another? What fears come up as you think of reaching or achieving your goal weight?

Ask yourself: What would it feel like to change?

What would it feel like for you to have achieved your weight loss goals? What would your life look like? Write out what it would be like to live a life where you put your health and happiness in front of the immediate gratification of a quick fix. Ask yourself: What might that feel like? What would it feel like to turn down food? What would it feel like to say no? What would it feel like to do things that are good for you? What would it feel like to eat bari-friendly meals? What would it feel like to use tools to help you manage your emotions? What would it feel like to get a hold on your stress?

Ask yourself: What does daily lifestyle change look like for you?

What steps in the bariatric basics would best serve you? How can you start small to gain traction to get back on track? What steps would you take? What does that look like? How does it feel? Is it freeing? Does it put you back in control? Do you feel powerful? What feelings come up?

Next Step: Take Action (This is your recommitment to yourself)

Do ONE thing to recommit to your journey—ONE step at a time.

This recommitment plan helps you to GET SUPER REAL with yourself. The only person sabotaging you IS YOU. The only person making you sick IS YOU. The only one who can SAVE you IS YOU.

I'm only here to empower you and help you put the power back in your hands... You may think you are powerless, but in fact, you are powerful. This journey is about getting healthy in more ways than one. You can do this; all you need is a little faith and elbow grease.

REFLECTION QUESTIONS

These are just a few of the questions I get when someone has lost their way and experienced regain after bariatric surgery.

1. What does recommitment look like?
2. What would I need to do?
3. How would I implement it?
4. Where do I begin?

THE RE-BEGINNING

Start where you are. Start Small. And just start. To reduce overwhelm or overthinking it, it must be simple. It begins with ONE meal. It begins with ONE workout. It begins with your decision to do something different. All it takes is ONE step.

You don't need to wait until Sunday or Monday. You just need to start today. Putting your "start date" off until next week, next Sunday or Monday, or another random day illustrates that you are not yet ready to begin.

You may need to go back and check-in with where you are in the stages of change. Many people are so afraid of giving something up that they procrastinate change and then get stuck in a cycle of being angry at themselves for "letting this happen," or for having regained the weight, and at the same time, are not completely ready to do the things, take action, and follow through with the CHANGE itself.

Does this sound like you?

Are you ready for a change?? Let's do this!

CHAPTER 2

Refocus on what you want

"You can't ride two horses with one ass, sugar bean."
— Sweet Home Alabama

What do you want to achieve?

What do you hope to gain from this process?

The truth is you likely have NO freaking idea what you want, and that my dear is the biggest problem of all. That's is likely the core of what's holding you back—this and shining object syndrome. I also refer to this as plan-hopping. Plan-hopping is when someone starts a plan, they do not stay on the plan long enough to see results. Instead, they "hop" on over to another plan hoping to get faster results. These individuals are typical "dieters," who want fast, quick results, which leads to confusion, self-doubt, frustration, and deprivation. Plan-hoppers go from one plan to the next so often, and it makes your head spin. Then they get frustrated when they don't see results. Then they get more frustrated when they cannot stick with anything.

Ohhh ... I should do weight watchers.

Oh no ... I need to do keto. I heard that one is faster.

Oh, wait ... I think I'll do paleo.

Well, on second thought, maybe I should just stick with low-carb.

It is not just food or meal plans that they plan-hop with. They do this with fitness too.

Ohh! Maybe I should do yoga, or what about Pilates?

Ohhh ... I heard high-intensity interval training is best.

A ton of people are doing CrossFit, and maybe I should do that. My friend Aileen says she's lost a ton of weight doing that. Maybe I will try that.

Plan hoppers also stay confused, which can trigger confusion, distraction, and self-doubt in other aspects of life as well.

Did someone just bring donuts into the office? Oooh, DONUTS! Wait ... do I want a donut, or don't I?

Oooh, a new position is open in my department. I wonder if I will get the promotion if I apply for it. Why would anyone pick me? Wait, do I even want it?

STOP.

BREATHE.

REFLECT.

Our culture right now is distracted, spread thin, and over-stimulated.

We have so much stimulus and so many competing priorities that we don't know if we're coming or going. You don't have to have a diagnosis for ADHD for this to be an issue. It's just happening as a result of daily life, social media, multi-tasking, and all the information that is presented to us on a daily basis.

It's overwhelming, and most often, we don't know where to turn.

Eat this, not that. No, do cardio. No, do CrossFit.

Multiple messages bombard you with not knowing where to turn or what to do. This might lead you to go back to dieting even if you thought surgery would change that. I frequently see individuals who go from diet to diet after bariatric surgery, hoping that the latest fad will change them, heal them, and finally keep the weight off.

Decision-making can be overwhelming, and what's even worse is flip-flopping from one diet to the next, from one decision to the next, not really committing to anything.

Not being committed to anything and being overcommitted to everything is a core issue. This brings to mind a saying, "How you do one thing is how you do everything." When you engage in a pattern to be uncommitted, confused, or unable to make a decision, that will start to show up in other areas of your life. The purpose here is not to beat you down, but to encourage you to change this pattern for your future.

By the way, it's not the diet that will heal you—it's YOU that will heal you. Let that sink in.

The solution you are seeking is inside of you. It's about shifting your perceptions around food. It's about recognizing WHY you eat and how to work through your emotions and behaviors. It's choosing to slow down and decide what you truly desire to create in your life. The solution is YOU. When you choose YOU, and when you become committed to you, no matter what, things begin to change. You begin to change.

CHOOSING YOU

The path to choosing you can be difficult and arduous because, for a long time, you may have been living for other people's desires, other people's intentions of you, or other people's expectations of you. If you are one of the select few that live life with self-intention, you are one step closer to uncovering the true you. Often in this weight loss journey, I meet men and women who have no clue who they are, what they want, or whom they want to become once they've lost the weight. This can be more difficult than the weight loss process itself because many try to fill in the gaps with other people's expectations of who they "should" be rather than asking using guidance from their own inner wisdom.

This post-operative process of lifestyle change goes beyond food and drink. It goes beyond what physical activity you engage in or how much sleep you get. It's about choosing you and creating a NEW you that emerges from this process.

Choosing you begins with acknowledging that you want to live differently from your former self. You had this surgery for a reason and for a life that you dreamed about living. Things you wanted to do that the weight had stood in your way for so long. This is the life that you get to create by choosing you.

The short-term need for immediate gratification may lead you to the food in the present, yet in the long-term, food takes you back to that old lifestyle you lived as a pre-op. Take this opportunity to practice mindfulness in the present to be more conscious of your food choices, so that you can put yourself back in control of your eating behaviors. You can reprogram your brain to respond differently. However, if you continue to condition the primitive limbic brain to rely on food as part of receiving pleasure, over time, you'll feel compelled, even driven, to have it. When food is in control, you are led back to the old coping mechanism and the old patterns. Getting clear with yourself on your desires can help you address what you want from your life beyond the food.

If food is the only thing you have that makes you happy, you can become stuck, because you will likely continue to go back to food to seek fulfillment and gratification. An important task for you now is to find other things that bring joy and happiness that aren't correlated with or connected to food. In my practice, I encounter many individuals grieving over food after weight loss surgery because they've lost one of their greatest sources of pleasure. This post-operative process is not about taking away pleasure, but about guiding you instead of toward a richer and more fulfilling life, separate from food. Don't let food be your focus. Instead, let YOU be your focus. Watch how things change when you focus on yourself, your happiness, and your desires.

DIGGING DEEPER INTO WHAT YOU TRULY WANT

Most people don't know what they want in their life. Despite having day-to-day functions, elements of dissatisfaction and unhappiness still emerge.

Often people can tell you what they dislike about their life, their current work situation, their relationships, and so on. However, when you ask them what they do want, they cannot tell you. Our brains can only filter through so much information at once. When faced with an unlimited supply of opportunities available to us, even to imagine, we are unable to comprehend it. It's like a computer overload; only it's happening to your brain. Your brain is your computer processor. So, rather than overloading the system by asking it a complex question that leaves it in a conundrum, you might start by being more specific, or you might start by working in reverse.

Instead of asking yourself what you truly want, you might make out a list of all the things that aren't working in your life or things you would like to release or get rid of in your life. You may look at all the disruptions, distractions, and things that make you unhappy. Look at the things that keep you stuck, frustrated, sad, and so on.

After you've listed out all the things you dislike about your life, then go through and see how you can take that situation, experience, event, etc., and flip it to something that you desire. Then work through how you might implement a plan to get that thing, situation, experience, relationship, event, etc.

Often, we make life so complex or much harder than it needs to be. In my previous book, *Bariatric Mindset Success*, I also encouraged people to find themselves and grow beyond their perceived limitations. I included a chapter on getting to know the new you. After weight loss surgery, many individuals are lost. They continue the life cycle that they created before surgery, and they are not the same person anymore. Can you imagine changing everything about how you look, but staying the same? That doesn't happen. We change. We evolve. We grow. However, if you don't figure out who that person is, and what they desire, the cycle of weight gain and weight loss may continue. And food will continue to be the central source of comfort, attention, distraction, and really the main source of everything. Getting out of this cycle begins with you getting to know yourself. It begins with you getting excited about living again. Living life again starts by recognizing what you are ready to release or let go of, and what you are ready to bring in or create for your life.

It may seem overwhelming at first, but trust me, it can be a mind-blowing process when you finally dig deep enough to recognize that you may have been settling this whole time. You deserve to live a life you are madly in love with. And the only person that can find out what that looks like, how that might feel, or what that experience will be like, is YOU.

Recently a client shared how unhappy she was since surgery. She was frustrated with her husband, her job, and her life. She realized something had to change. She started to dig deeper into what she wanted, which began with her reflecting on what was working and not working in her life. She reflected on all her struggles, including the ones that led her back to food as a coping mechanism. She made her list of things she wanted to release and started to think about what she wanted to create for her life. Not too long after she conducted this activity with me, and begin to reflect on her journey, she was offered a huge opportunity at work. It was through this opportunity that she was able to move her family cross country, which is something her husband had been bugging her about for months. This promotion and move have led her to greater fulfillment, which has impacted her weight journey as well. Her focus changed to other areas of her life, which left food as a source of nourishment, rather than a pastime she used to soothe her unraveling emotions.

In life, we must put our focus and attention back on the real problems in order that we can achieve happiness, success, and fulfillment. When we seek to solve our problems by using food to cope with the problems, we only get bigger, and as a result, we create bigger problems.

Finding who you are and what you want is a great starting point for this journey. Reflecting on where you've been and where you want to go can also help you recognize that staying the same will only lead you back to the same old patterns.

Change the pattern of your questions to help you shift the focus back to you.

Ask yourself, what do I dislike in my life?

Then ask, what would I like to create instead?

Let's take a deep dive into you. Are you ready? Buckle up, and let's go.

REFLECTION QUESTIONS

1. What are the things you like to do with friends and family?
2. How many of these activities are centered around food?
3. What activities would you like to engage in that do not revolve around food?
4. What would you do with your life if there were limitless possibilities?
5. What have you always dreamed of doing in your life but haven't yet?
6. What would be a game-changer for you in your life?
7. What would you like to see your day-to-day life be like? Where would you go? What would you do? Whom would you see?
8. If you allowed yourself to let go of fear, who would you become?
9. If you allowed yourself to live beyond fear, who would you be?
10. If you allowed yourself to live your best life, what would that look like? Who would you share it with? Where would you live? What would you do? Whom would you be? What would your passion be? What would change for you?

11. What is holding you back from achieving any or all of this now?
12. What limitations do you hold in your mind that says you "can't" be, do, or have any of these things you desire.
13. Write out your ideal day. What would you do from start to finish? Who would you see, where would you go, what would you do?

If these reflection questions and journaling prompts are not enough to help you uncover your desires, take a look at my *Rediscover You Journal*, available on Amazon, which includes an additional 75 self-discovery journaling prompts aimed at helping you get to the core you.

CHAPTER 3

Recommit to the Basics

Remember, in chapter 1, when I asked you what "back on track" looked like for you? We're going to take your adjusted definition of *back on track* and use that to help guide you to a lasting lifestyle change. When you recommit to being back on track and the basics, you're recommitting to taking consistent action for YOU. In this chapter, I'm going to take a moment to go over the basics. Then I'll focus on how you recommit to them.

I also want to take this time to scream and shout from the top of my lungs, "For the love of God, stop going from one diet to the next and back again!" I firmly believe this ONE thing is keeping you stuck the most. And, the diet industry LOVES you.

You had bariatric surgery, and you have an amazing tool at your disposal. Let's use it to your advantage. There is no short cut to a lifestyle change. Diets will always be out there, and they will inevitably lead you back here. Part of our work together is to banish diets and help you to heal your relationship with food. This means back to basics and starting over using your tools. This does NOT mean using pouch resets.

The pouch will mess with your mind just like a diet will, and you'll feel depleted and deprived. Back to basics is so much better for you than attempting to go back to a fully liquid diet.

Many swear by resets, and I bet that those individuals end up in a cycle of regaining and reset. You're here because you want to lose the regain and weight for good, not get stuck in a cycle of regain only to need to reset.

Not to mention that only a small part of the population would be able to sustain this for six days anyway without really struggling mentally. I see people all the time struggling with pre-op liquid diets. It is likely similar post-op as well.

This process isn't a diet. This is a lifestyle change.

And, the whole reason you started on liquids to begin with after surgery was so your stomach could heal effectively.

Leaving the *diet* behind, stopping the reset madness, and practicing lifestyle change will get you farther faster. Repeating the diet cycle ensures you also continue the gain/loss cycle, not to mention keeping you frustrated.

If you return to eating full-fat fried chicken and biscuits weekly, I guarantee beyond a shadow of a doubt, and you will regain your weight.

If you eat donuts daily...

If you run through the drive-through daily...

If you fill your body with the chemically-laden foods, for the sake of convenience...

What do you honestly think will happen by repeating old patterns?

It all repeats a cycle that you want to leave behind. And if you're struggling, let go of any destructive habits, you may need deeper work, and that's okay.

No, I'm not the food police—but I am blunt and honest. And I wholeheartedly believe if I don't keep it real with you, I won't be speaking with integrity.

If someone goes back to Doritos, Coke, and fast food on a daily or even weekly basis, it's a recipe for disaster.

And, I see it in my community ... ALL ... THE ... TIME ...

I know the excuses—all of them.

I know how busy you are.

I work with the overworked single moms on a limited budget.

I work with the traveling professionals who go in and out of the airport constantly.

I work with the men who have two jobs trying to make ends meet for their families.

I work with retirees that have the time but can't get themselves to cook.

I work with the high achievers who would rather work themselves up the corporate ladder than getting stuck in the kitchen for an hour.

I see you all. I know you all. I feel the pain you endure.

And here you are. Struggling.

The BASICS are here to guide you back to you, not to limit you.

They are meant to help you expand your life, not deplete it.

And yet, you haven't figured out how to work the basics into your lifestyle.

So, I'm going to teach you.

But first, I want to remind you: I am not the food person. I'm the mindset person.

What does this mean??

This means I don't give out meal plans. I'm not that person. For all those that say, "I don't know what to eat," I have to call you out and call BULLSHIT. The number of classes that are given on nutrition in this community is astounding. The amount of social media pages and groups on cooking and healthy eating is again ... ASTOUNDING!!

They are everywhere. So, I call ... BS!

You can get angry. You can throw this book down. You can get upset.

And if someone is reading this that legitimately does NOT know what to eat, reach out to me on Facebook, and I'll connect you with a variety of nutritional resources that will help you guide you with eating. My point here is that 'what to eat' is not the main issue. It's only a symptom of the issue, and it's one that is keeping you confused.

You DO know what to eat. Saying you don't is your way of clinging to confusion and preventing you from actually starting to get back on track. Because, if you don't know what to eat, then you don't have to start ...

RIGHT?

Even if you had surgery overseas or in countries that provide zero, zilch, nada nutrition counseling, I bet you still would know what to eat.

High Protein.

Low Carb.

Fresh Vegetables.

Low Glycemic Index Fruit.

Water.

Most of us could write a book on nutrition, so I'm not buying the "I don't know what to eat" line.

This is an excuse that keeps you from starting.

DOZENS of keto, high protein, low-carb, and bariatric friendly recipes can be found on Pinterest and all over the internet. The truth is, I know that many of you know what to eat and how to eat. Many Instagram pages, Facebook groups, Pinterest pages, and sites are dedicated to bariatric friendly foods. A lack of information on WHAT to eat is not the issue. That is for sure.

If you're telling me you don't know what to eat? I doubt it.

Maybe you don't know how to pull it all together, or to make it easy. Or, you get frustrated because cooking is not your thing.

Please stop telling yourself you don't know what to eat.

When I was starting out as a patient, one of the techs at my surgical center gave some great advice. She said, "You can eat the inside of a sandwich (avoid the bread), you can grab some lunch meat and cheese, and, BAM, you have lunch." She shared that we could order the protein from just about any restaurant and make it a healthy choice.

At one of my nutrition classes, the nurse suggested we bought a prepared rotisserie chicken from the grocery store when we were in a rush. Pair it with a vegetable, and, BAM, you have a meal. This does not have to be hard. It really doesn't.

So why are people so confused about what to eat?

Being confused about what to eat keeps you stuck in confusion, as I noted above. Why would anyone WANT to stay in confusion? See, if you don't know how to change, then you wouldn't know how to take action on it either. Or, if you are committed or addicted to fast foods, high-fat foods, fried foods, you may decide to stay in this pattern to avoid dealing with it.

Some people don't want to have to give up their convenience foods. Some people don't want to make difficult changes. Some people aren't ready for change. Some people want to avoid what is uncomfortable, and change is uncomfortable. And then, there are those that have a rebellious streak— "You can't tell me what to do."

You know who you are.

While all this may seem harsh, hear me out. Another part of this pattern is emotional eating. Avoiding healthy foods can be a pattern of dealing with emotional pain. Not wanting to invest in yourself, take a chance on you, heal the trauma, or deal with the emotional pain can be a cycle in itself.

Individuals who have experienced trauma don't know what it's like to be healthy or whole. They may cling to an experience that is all they knew to help them, to soothe them, to make them feel normal. This may have been food. And to take this food away can be traumatizing. To avoid further trauma, to avoid losing their coping mechanism, they go with what they know, and as a result, they return to old patterns.

For others, they may begin to eat healthy for a while, and then return to seeking out the old foods that soothe their emotional needs.

With this book, I want to help you adjust to the psychology piece and implement the changes.

WHAT ARE THE BASICS?

1. **Eat protein first at meals.**

   Protein is the priority. It is a building block to gaining muscle and helps you stay full longer. This is a nutrition recommendation of the ASMBS (American Society of Metabolic and Bariatric Surgery).

2. **Move your body regularly.**

   Movement helps you to produce endorphins, which make you feel better and improves your mood. It also helps your body to become an efficient calorie-burning machine. A ton of research suggests the movement is great for your brain, your mood, and your body. It's not about weight loss as much as it is for health.

3. **Drink water. Get at least 64oz of water per day.**

   Drinking water helps you to flush toxins from your body and helps you to flush fat during your WLS journey.

4. **Take your vitamins and supplements.**

   Most bariatric patients are at risk for nutrient deficiency, so it is important to take your doctor-recommended supplements. Bariatric-friendly vitamins are the best to ensure you're getting the right dosage. Regular over-the-counter vitamins typically don't have the recommended dose to support the needs of a bariatric patient. Vitamins/supplements support your weight loss process. Vitamin deficiencies like Vitamin D and Vitamin B can impact your energy, leaving you lethargic. Several other vitamin deficiencies can also impact your health.

5. **Get plenty of sleep.**

   Not sleeping enough is another major factor in weight regain. Sleep is of vital importance for your body to recover from day-to-day activities. Not getting enough sleep can impact your body's functioning. The recommendations are typically 6-8 hours of sleep per night. Studies show that individuals who do not get enough sleep are at risk of eating 400+ more calories per day in an attempt to keep themselves awake. Eating to "keep going" is a way for your body and brain to trigger the neurotransmitter dopamine that impacts motivation. Ever go for a 3 pm pick-me-up snack or coffee because you needed to "push through"? If this is a struggle for you, contact your doctor, and get a sleep study.

OTHER BASIC GUIDELINES

Eat ONLY at mealtimes and avoid grazing.

What's grazing? And why should I avoid it?

Grazing is known as the behavior of eating or snacking arbitrarily between meals and when not physically hungry. Grazing can create head hunger, eating as a habit, and weight gain. Head hunger or habitual hunger occurs when someone eats at the same time every day and has created eating as a habit. If someone grazes daily at 3 pm or 9 pm, their brain may expect to continue to eat at that time. They may not be physically hungry but instead have a desire to eat at these times because they have programmed themselves to expect to eat then. Grazing should be avoided because it typically leads to emotional eating rather than utilizing one's hunger cues. Grazing can also be synonymous with mindless eating and/or bored eating.

And remember – NO eating and drinking within 30-min of one another.

Why?

Because the smaller pouch or sleeve created after surgery is not large enough to sustain both food and liquids at the same time. Additionally, liquids can push food through the pouch faster, which then leads to a disruption in fullness and hunger cues. Waiting before and after eating can help individuals feel satiated, so they feel hungry less often.

Many of these issues have been covered in greater detail in my first book, *Bariatric Mindset Success: Keep the Weight Off and Live Your Best Life after Bariatric Surgery*. For more tools and insight on the basics, be sure to check this out and add it to your bariatric library.

OTHER NUTRITIONAL INSIGHT

Like I've said before, I'm not the nutrition expert, I'm the mindset expert. However, I do know and will cite my sources to support the following knowledge.

After working with so many women over the years, I've learned we all have different nutritional needs. For example, some people do better eating a balanced macros plan. While many balanced plans suggest 50% carbs, 25% protein, and 25% fat, the nutrition research suggests that the average bariatric patient needs to adjust that to eat lower carbs and higher protein. This modifies the macros to a net balance of 35% carbohydrates, 40% protein, and 25% fat. The nutritionist that I work with has had incredible success helping individuals on a balanced macros plan, which helps many reach their weight loss goal and live comfortably in maintenance. Others do better to keep their weight off with a higher protein, lower-carbohydrate plan. Some do even better with an adjusted keto-type plan.

The nutrition research suggests that people who struggle with insulin resistance do well practicing living with low-carbohydrate plans after weight loss surgery. Studies support that those who have Polycystic

Ovarian Syndrome (PCOS) do better on a variation of the ketogenic plan, dirty keto, lazy keto, or the like (Galletly, et al., 2007; Russa, 2019).

While bariatric surgery can help with PCOS and insulin resistance, the research suggests that these issues don't just go away. Therefore, these patients do better post-operatively on a very low-carbohydrate plan like a keto plan to keep the weight off. These plans also combat sugar cravings and help maintain weight loss. I've seen women with those medical conditions move to this behavioral and nutritional change time and time again and have greater success than on any other plan. If you are concerned about which plan is the best fit for you, be sure to consult with your own nutrition provider or connect with me on social media, and I'll connect you with a certified nutritionist.

MANAGING LIFE STRESSORS

Life stressors can lead to emotional eating or off-track eating. Typically, life and/or emotional stressors create behavioral change in individuals. The reason could be one of many. Whether it is a job change or a fear of a job loss, stressors may create anxiety or tension in one's life. An impending divorce or the loss of a parent or loved one creates stress. Whatever the case may be, dealing with stress can impact your ability to eat healthily. If you end up throwing your hands up in the air and taking care of everyone or everything else but yourself, it will end up showing up in your life one way or another.

Taking care of your basic needs, such as nutrition and movement, are essential for both your mental and physical wellness. Putting it off or avoidance only leads to greater discontent.

While everyone is bound to experience life stressors, these circumstances are not final or fatal. Working through them offers an opportunity to get beyond them. Accountability, having a support system, and even attending counseling or therapy, is important during this time. Everyone is not expected to have a full toolbox ready to deal with life stressors when they strike. Learning to manage stress is one of the most important tools for the post-operative bariatric lifestyle.

REFLECTION QUESTIONS

1. What can I begin to do today to take care of me?
2. What does the term *self-care* mean to me?
3. What do '*commit to the basics* and *back on track*' mean for me in my weight loss journey?
4. How can I apply simple practices daily that is back on track while implementing the basics?
5. What are the basics that I resist committing to on my journey?
6. What are the basics that I'm willing to commit to this week?
7. What is one small step I can take today?
8. What can I do to change my thinking about the basics so I can be more successful long-term?
9. What are the emotional stressors that most impact my ability to follow through with the basics?
10. What can I do to address those emotional or life stressors?
11. What barriers do I have toward meal planning or meal prepping?

CHAPTER 4

Reprioritize Your Process

On this journey, I see so many people struggling with the process, their mindset, how to change, and all the difficulties and barriers they perceive as they move along.

By no means am I suggesting this is an easy journey; however, there are a few ways to make it easier.

Scientific studies suggest that when you add the element of play or fun to challenging situations, they FEEL easier even if they aren't. So why not play with it?

Let's make it fun!

You might be thinking, *What do you mean, make it fun? How will this stuff ever be fun?*

OH, yes, it can be fun. Have you ever danced in your living room? Put on some heart-pumping music and just danced? See, this is FUN!

Moving your body can be fun.

When you do things that make you feel good, it creates ease and positive emotions. If you only see moving your body as something painful or unsatisfying, then it will be. Creating fun and ease in your movement routine will help you implement it as part of lasting lifestyle change. We do things that are fun and easy. We avoid doing things that are difficult or hard. Similarly, if you tell yourself that fitness is hard and takes too long, then you'll likely avoid it. If you tell yourself it is fun and easy, you will likely follow through. Your belief system runs the show here.

SHIFT YOUR PERSPECTIVE

A few years ago, a client told me, "I'm not the kind of person who works out." She then proceeded to tell me she disliked sweating, and she disliked going to the gym. She shared it made her feel uncomfortable. Initially, we worked on her belief system, which helped her to shift her perspective around movement. Her deep-seated belief about movement, physical activity, and "working out" came from the pain she experienced due to her extra weight. Following her surgery and her 138-pound weight loss, her body moved easier, but her belief about the movement was still present. Initially, I asked her about her other beliefs, which helped her see how this belief about movement had held her back.

In our work, we focused on how the behavior would help her, rather than her focus on what she was avoiding. In her mind, the exercise was painful, even after she had lost the weight. This attitude was reflected in her belief system. We worked on creating alternate thoughts about exercise to help her develop a new belief system about physical activity. We also worked through the logic she had created in order to break it down.

I started by asking her about other activities that were healthy that she was already doing. We discussed other activities, such as brushing her teeth or washing her hands. I joked with her, "Well if I'm not the kind of person who brushes their teeth, I wouldn't have any teeth." We then used this example as a way to unravel her core beliefs about other things. She then went on to use the example of work, stating, "If I'm not the type of person who 'works,' I would imagine that I'd also have a hard time supporting myself." In the end, we had a good chuckle because it made sense. This belief pattern was what she had been using to justify not moving her body, which has many health benefits. She was also so used to not moving that she had an old limiting belief programmed that it would hurt, even when it didn't hurt anymore. In the end, we got her moving!

Here's the thing we uncovered at the core of it all: PERSPECTIVE.

These changes were all mindset! Her past core beliefs, along with her unrealistic perspective, kept her stuck. In shifting her perspective, she was able to find activities that were fun, stimulating, and exciting to move her body. She even created a weekly routine that included dance, swimming, and yoga. The point here is not WHAT you do because you can choose from a plethora of activities, only that you shift your mindset to change your patterns of behavior, which can positively impact your health.

The limitations occur as a result of how you perceive difficulties, and the results come from your ability to overcome them from within your mind's eye.

Wayne Dyer said, "*When you change the way you look at things, the things you look at change.*"

Meaning, that when you change your perspective or your outlook, you can create a different result.

If you consistently look at things in your life as a chore, they will be. However, if you begin to look at things as part of your journey, you may see them as far less daunting than when you saw them as a chore. It's all perspective, and of course, **#mindset**.

Similarly, the person committed to their long-term health recognizes that relying on willpower in the present is not feasible and can be problematic. This is because willpower is not sustainable. Discipline is needed over willpower, and discipline is all about scheduling and planning.

Planning ahead, meal prepping, and working out, are all part of the healthy routine needed to achieve one's goal weight and maintain that goal weight as part of lifestyle change. However, one of the trends I've seen over the years within the bariatric community, and those struggling with obesity (yes, including myself and my own patterns over the years as a pre-op!), has been the amount of overwhelm, experienced day-in and day-out. They've run themselves ragged, which then leads them to a lifestyle of needing the "quick and easy," which tends to be the same road leading to weight struggles.

Everyone seems to think this is due to laziness, but it is more due to a lack of life skills, not laziness like everyone seems to think. The old survival mechanism is to rush, rush, rush, and then rest. Rush, rush, rush ... and then ... REST. See the problem with this pattern?

The problem with that line of thinking is that you end up "cutting off your nose to spite your face," meaning that time is spent on activities that may not create an impact or reward you on your journey. The new mindset shift line of thinking is, "let me plan ahead and get this done, to enjoy my downtime later."

Another helpful line of thinking is to make meal planning and meal prep part of your new lifestyle. In this same line of thinking, moving your body or fitness (whichever you choose to refer to it), becomes part of your new lifestyle. It's not extra. It's not a drag. It is part of living a healthy life. However, if you're thinking of it as something you *have* to do, rather than something that comes with this new lifestyle, then yes, you'll make it harder on yourself.

Once again, though, I know it is an adjustment to an already busy life. Creating time in your day to prioritize these activities as *important* is essential to losing weight regain and entering maintenance. If these things are not part of your plan, it will be more difficult to get to the goal.

The thought pattern and mindset shifts are needed because the emotional connection to food (what feels good) and the overwhelm or exhaustion of daily life may come from being overweight for a long period of time or may come from other habits, such as overworking, people-pleasing, and doing for others rather than setting healthy boundaries, making time for prepping/planning and practicing self-care.

Taking care of yourself goes beyond making doctors' appointments, it also includes preventative care. In order to prevent illness, the focus must be on wellness. In order to create wellness, wellness must be prioritized. Yet in the busyness of life, people are often chasing their own tails, allowing life to become cycles of overdoing in some areas and underdoing in others.

Another quotation useful here is, "Before cutting your neighbor's grass, work on your own."

This state of life calls for greater balance overall. Yet, so many resist the balance because of the greater stimulus in the hustle-bustle of living an overwhelmed life than one of planning and preparation. I find that most people are so addicted to *busy* that they don't make room for priorities such as planning and prepping. They thrive on chaos because that's all they have ever known. Others find it boring to plan or prep and tend to avoid it because they perceive it as more work. Then they lump it into a "work" category, making it low on the priority list.

If the perception were that planning and prepping could save you time, money, headaches, and the extra weight, would the mindset change or stay the same?

If you knew that by restructuring your time to be more efficient and effective could actually save you time and provide for your health, would you do it?

What is important to recognize is that some small life hacks can create big results and big change when implemented over time.

And, it's essential that your thoughts about these activities shift to focusing on what will help you instead of feeling resistant to change or being fixated on what's uncomfortable.

All change, no matter the size, can be uncomfortable because it's not the norm—it's outside your typical routine. This fact is important to remember, regardless of what you are implementing.

You also must recognize whether or not you are emotionally resisting regular day-to-day tasks. Tasks are not emotional; they are just tasks. However, I see many people who go straight to "I don't want to," and this keeps them stuck.

If your boss asked you to do something you'd wouldn't likely respond with, "I don't want to," yet, when it comes to your own self-care, health, and wellness, "I don't want to" becomes an option. When you make your wellness something that you must be in the MOOD for, you make it optional instead of something you just DO. This mindset makes the difference between those who have created a disciplined practice and those who consistently struggle. This is because discipline is about learning. Even the root of the word "discipline" comes from the Latin root "*to study*". Therefore, discipline is about learning, studying, practicing, and engaging consistently in a new way of BEING.

Making lifestyle change a part of your life differs from making it a choice. If it is an option and you don't have to cook a healthy dinner, then you don't. If it is an option whether or not to move your body or workout, then you might not. But when it is a standard of living for health, when it is a non-negotiable for a healthy lifestyle, it's just something you do, not something you debate in your mind.

Similarly, when it is a standard of care for yourself, you know exactly when you act on it in your life. When it is an option, you try to figure out "where to fit it in." It's either something you prioritize as an essential part of life to be healthy, and it's consistent. Or, it's something you "might do," which then can fall to the bottom of the list when life gets busy.

This is the stark difference between the thought process.

Do you see the difference?

How do you want to live your life? As the main character of your story or as a walk-on actor that may or may not contribute to the story? This analogy may be how you are living your life. It's not just the weight regain that is freaking you out – it's all the stuff that goes with it.

In order to lose weight, it's not just the behaviors that need to change. It's you and your mindset about the behaviors that also needs to change.

ACTIVITY: BREAK IT DOWN

Breaking tasks down into smaller chunks can help with reducing overwhelm. Often, I hear people say, "When am I supposed to get it all done?" The truth is, you can get it all done when you break it down into smaller chunks.

Here are some examples of breaking tasks down into smaller, doable chunks that help to save time and energy.

- Turn all-day meal prep into two or three 30-min or 1-hour time blocks.
- Chop all your veggies needed for meal prep, and this may take 20 minutes.
- Conduct a 10-minute dish-dash where you wash your dishes and put them in the dishwasher while you have music playing.
- Conduct a 5- or 10-minute decluttering segment, where you focus on one section of one room in your house.
- Go for a 10-minute walk or lift weights for the same amount of time to fit in your fitness routine.

The point here is: You can squeeze things into your day without requiring larger chunks of time to get them done.

ACTIVITY: MAKE IT EASY

In one of my online groups, I challenged participants to reframe their mindset on something they originally associated with being "hard" to something they can make "easy."

For context, a few shared that getting to the gym and working out was hard for them, while others shared that their hardest tasks were meal prep, folding clothes, emptying the dishwasher, or other household tasks.

As a result, we created a new thought process that helped them to make it easy.

See, when you repeat to yourself in your head over and over and over that something is hard, you believe it. This becomes your foundational belief system, and you believe it as truth. Then, it truly becomes hard. You feel the weight of the emotion you've created in your mind, and it comes into your reality. It becomes hard, and then it becomes painful. It becomes so hard that you avoid it. You don't do it. You procrastinate. And then, you don't follow through. Ever.

Let's do an experiment. Go for a quick walk—5 minutes—and the entire time talks to yourself about how hard the walk is, how your feet hurt, how you have so many other things to do but walk, how it's difficult, and you don't want to, and really make an impact with your self-talk. Make it hard!! Repeat over and over to yourself about how hard and difficult it is. And record on a sheet of paper how "hard" this experience felt for you on a scale of 1-10.

Now, go for that same 5-minute walk, talking differently about your experience. Instead, now label the walk as easy. Talk it up in your head. Change the monologue in your mind: *This is so easy. I can do this. Wow, I am almost there. This feels so good, and it is so easy. This is much easier than I believed it to be.* Maybe even laugh about how easy it is. Share how easy it is for you to walk for this time. "Wow, almost there. So close! Only a few more yards. Is this really 5 minutes? We are almost done. This is so easy. I could do this every day. Walking is so easy." Really talk up the ease. Now, go back to that paper and evaluate the ease on a scale of 1-10.

Here is my point: If you want to make it easy, you can. If you want to make it harder, you can. It all starts within your mind. You'll notice that how you think about things can make them harder or easier, based on your perspective.

ACTIVITY: TIME-SAVING HACKS

Prioritizing Meal Prep – Successful weight loss maintainers make meal prep a priority. You might break this down into two- or three-time blocks in order to fit it into your schedule. It does not have to take up your entire weekend, although many people prefer to conduct meal-prep on weekends. Schedule an hour or so on your calendar two to three days per week to make your meals. This will ensure you have healthy meals at your fingertips and aren't rushing out to grab fast food. Making extra servings, you can put in your freezer will also save you time. One of my clients makes protein balls and egg muffins once a month and freezes them for easy on-the-go breakfasts.

Scheduling Workouts – Schedule your workouts just like you would a doctor's appointment. Put it on your schedule and commit to that day and time. Maybe you'll just be walking the dog, or playing a YouTube workout, or maybe you do have a gym commitment. Regardless of what it is, following through on time on your calendar will keep you more accountable.

Timing Your Activities – Whether you are doing household chores, decluttering, paying bills, or running errands, time yourself. Make it a game where you time yourself and how long it will take to get it done. Many of my clients are exhausted by the things they have to do, and as a result, they avoid their day-to-day responsibilities. When they use a timer to time themselves, they find that they get things done faster and with less emotion involved. The tasks are just tasks, nothing else. They get them done, and they move on with their day. However, the time they previously invested in deciding what they wanted to do when they had delayed getting the activity completed, which ended up making them more miserable and frustrated. The "just do it" mentality helps you to time yourself, take action, and get it done.

ACTIVITY: REMOVING THE EMOTION

When we give emotion to tasks, we make them weigh more in our minds. If you are loathing doing a specific task because you hate it, you have just added "hate weight" to the task. You've made it harder instead of easier.

To change this, allow a task to be a task. Stop giving it emotional attention. So, let's say you hate going to the gym. Instead of making the gym an emotional decision, put it in your mind just like you would a trip to get gas, or buy groceries or run any other errand. It's just something that has to get done. It's just part of that routine. When you demonize it, when your emotions get in the way, you avoid doing it because you have deemed it unpleasant and optional.

Try these activities for about three months and see how much it changes your life, your habits, your weight, and your wellbeing.

One of my clients reported that she has been doing this with all of her previously labeled "hard" activities for about three months, and as a result, meal prepping and planning are a breeze, house chores are doable, and she's working out regularly. All because she told herself it was easy, removed the emotion from the equation, and followed through with her tasks.

REFLECTION QUESTIONS

1. When you did the walking exercise, what did you notice? Did you see the difference in how the walk felt for you? Did you notice a difference in your emotional state? Did you notice a difference in the level of ease when you focused on it?

2. Take your hardest tasks (or the ones you perceive as your most difficult tasks) and look for ways to make them easier. They may legitimately be difficult. Then talk to yourself in a way that helps you to make it easy. Create a timeline or schedule for yourself to get this done—set goals. Make a plan. Then take action. You might even keep a record of how much easier it gets over time.

3. Where would you like to create EASE in your life?

4. What are you willing to play with or make FUN in your life?

5. What can you shift the perspective on in your life?

6. What activities have been the hardest for you to complete or engage in?
7. What are you willing to prioritize for your health?
8. How can you change your perspective on tasks, from *have to*'s to get *to's* or *want to*'s and required essentials and basics on your weight loss journey?
9. What can you put into place to help you see these tasks differently?

CHAPTER 5

Restart Daily

We are what we repeatedly do.
Excellence, then, is not an act but a habit. – Aristotle

Your restart does not have to be this big overture where you wait until Monday, next weekend, or next January. Restarting is about being better every single day. It's about taking your basics and putting them into a routine. It's about taking action DAILY.

Build consistency with the basics, and you'll see that your life becomes easier. Instead of changes being a chore, they become part of your habits. When you commit to habits consistently, they become your lifestyle. Your lifestyle creates your results.

Your DAILY restart makes a difference.

Maybe you find it boring? Or maybe your excuse is "busyness," or maybe you're not stimulated enough to build this consistency.

However, in order to build consistency, you've got to START somewhere, and that somewhere is always DAY 1.

While the BASICS are a foundation of sorts, restarting daily helps you recognize that you have a fresh start every day.

This can be great for people who freak out about perfectionism, or it can be difficult for those who say, "Ehh, I can start tomorrow."

This is because the perfectionists are stuck in a cycle of 100% or 0%. So, for those of you who are perfectionists, I encourage you to give up the need for acquiring 100% of things because this is the key to your failure, not your success. Every personal and professional success story begins with failure, effort, and trying again—every single one!

Why would you think your path would be any different?

It's not. You may have heard the clichés and sayings like, "Each and every day is a clean slate and a fresh start." Maybe you gloss over phrases like this. Maybe you ignore them because you are so committed to the old patterns that you deny that you can restart. Or maybe you are still so busy punishing yourself for your missteps that you can't seem to let them go. Whatever the reason that you hold contempt, anger, frustration, or fear, it's time to let it go. The continued punishment of eating off track, failing once again, or giving in to temptation and then blaming or guilting yourself is part of that old pattern that leads you back to weight regain, not weight loss. This old pattern is the reason you are here. This old mindset of having to punish and hold yourself in contempt is NOT about accountability. It's about shame. Shame doesn't help you lose weight; in fact, it likely causes you to escape with food even more. When you're living in your old pattern of behaviors, you're more likely to say "screw it" after you've had that donut during your team's weekly meeting, causing you to maybe eat a couple more or eat something else triggering. The reasons are twofold. In your mind's eye, you've already messed up, so why not go for broke. Second, if you've already messed up today, you then give yourself permission to make good use of the "off track" day. You've already messed up today, so you will start over tomorrow. It's always putting things off until tomorrow. And, this, my friends, is the continued pattern that keeps you stuck. Instead of calling yourself out, allow compassion for the one stinking donut. You fly off the rails and then boom—an event about which you could have practiced forgiveness and compassion, instead becomes this catastrophic event that makes you feel a complete loss of self-control, along with a wave of shame, blame, guilt, and a whole-hell-of-a-lot of negative self-talk. Your negative inner critic has a field day during these moments. And then, just like that, you feel like a complete and utter failure. This old pattern can lead to weight regain because of the pain and frustration that is experienced over and over again. What is the behavior the makes you feel better? What is the thing you do to release yourself from feeling awful after a misstep happens? Often, the next behavior is more of the same, eating off track, which leads to cyclical patterns. Over time, this one pattern leads to weight regain. Then you blame yourself for not having control, but it's not about controlling yourself as much as practicing awareness in order to dissect the pattern, which then leads to making different choices. Taking back control of your mind and behaviors begins when you decide to see things differently, practice things differently, and get honest with yourself about the patterns in your life. What patterns are running the show? Which patterns do you fall into or choose? Which patterns can you learn from?

You are not bad. Food is not bad. The pattern is not bad. This is all subjective, and the story you've been telling about it may be what is making you feel worse. Instead of telling the old story and living the old patterns, you get to create a change. Just like professional athletes replay tapes in their off days to learn from their plays, you can, too! The quarterback that threw the interception last week is learning from that this week. The basketball player that got the ball knocked out of his hand right before he could have made the winning shot is learning from that today. You are no different. This process is no different. You can learn from everything that you are going through. It is constantly teaching you if you are willing to learn from it, and from this, you can change it.

The most important thing to recognize here: You have a choice. Instead of falling down that rabbit hole, you have an opportunity to choose differently. You can change the narrative and the story in your head. You can change the behaviors after the event. You can release the "donut" (or whatever you ate) incident, practice compassion, forgiveness, encouragement, and love, which will lead you to get back on track that same day. You can decide to get yourself back on track that same hour. You can decide that the donut doesn't mean as much as you think it does. You can decide that it doesn't mean failure, but that it is instead a learning experience, something you can gain insight from. You can decide that the "donut" doesn't represent failure, but instead represents an unmet need within you. You can look beyond the "donut" (or whatever it was), in order to shift your behavior in the direction you want it to be, rather than continuing the negative cycle that begets more off the rails eating, instead of less. You can learn from everything, and you can grow beyond it.

Restarting daily, or even hourly is important to adopt because it incorporates the mindset of recognizing that yesterday and tomorrow have no power. Tomorrow will not be the magic bullet to eating on track.

You have no idea what is going to happen tomorrow; yet, so many places their power there. Furthermore, there is no power in 5 minutes ago. There is no power in an hour ago. It's gone. It's over. It's done.

Today is the ONLY day you have power. This moment is the only moment you have power. The moment of your choices, and the moment of your decisions is where your power lies. The moment that you take action is the moment you wield your power. I hope to guide you to be here more often – in the PRESENT.

This moment is the ONLY moment you have power because you are making choices to do something FOR yourself, or you're making choices that go against what you SAY you want. Yesterday is gone; there is no power there. What you did yesterday is just a memory. Tomorrow hasn't come, and you cannot give your power to tomorrow, because you are not there yet. Your only power is in what you do today.

Like Yoda says, *"Do or do not, there is no try."*

Each and every day, you have an opportunity to shift gears to a new way of being. Procrastination actually keeps you stuck and strips you of your power.

Busyness is not an excuse. Believe me, I've worked with some of the busiest people, and I, myself, am a busy person. Busy does not give you a golden pass. You can live this lifestyle, regardless. It does not matter what you have going on. It is a mindset issue if you are not taking care of yourself. Even in the worst life situations, you can use mindset hacks to implement small, subtle shifts that create a lifestyle change.

I have worked with some of the busiest people with the craziest of schedules, and you can always find time for things that are important to you.

In fact, one of my mentors used to tell me, "You have exactly the amount of time and money for things that are important to you." She said, "If you want something really badly, you'll find the money to make it happen, and if you want to achieve something, you'll create the time in your day to make sure you do it."

Another quote that made sense, "You'll find the way, or you'll find an excuse."

Maybe you have seen one of those posts on social media about investments of money and time. They blew my mind, and I knew I had to share similar examples in our community. A few examples:

- A $100 dinner out is acceptable, but $100 in groceries is too expensive.
- A $40 per month gym membership is steep, but $40 per month on cable is cheap.
- A $50 bottle of diet pills is doable, but a $50 monthly healthy meal plan is expensive.
- A $30 wine bottle of the month club is doable, but $30 a month to invest in your education/wellness is ludicrous.
- A $200 program to move toward your health is pricey, but $200 on a new purse or pair of shoes is a must-have.

Do you see the pattern here?

The issues are in perspective and in the priorities. When you prioritize other things over your health and wellbeing, you are not valuing your health. People say they want to improve, but do they want to put in the work? Or are they afraid that it will cause pain or angst?

Our brains are hardwired for the pleasure/pain principle. We avoid pain and seek out pleasure. This principle is easily seen in the priorities listed above. While a person may state that health is a priority, people often have a perspective that it's HARD to live healthily. This perception is simply not true. It's just a perspective and a belief that people cling to. This false perspective is what makes it a mindset issue. The good news is it can be shifted, and it doesn't have to be as hard as you think it is!

As we discussed in the previous chapter, if you consistently repeat that you believe something will be hard, it will be hard, and you'll avoid it. On the other hand, if you work on creating ease, repeating to yourself that this can be easy, and you can do it, then you will. It's all in your mind. It's in what you tell yourself, and what belief you have on repeat.

The author and motivational speaker, Hal Elrod, is a perfect example of this. In his book, *The Miracle Morning*, Hal talks about his near-fatal car accident and his own journey back to health. He was told he would never walk again. Yet, he chose to believe differently. He worked on his mindset and has gone on to become an ultramarathon runner, keynote speaker, and world-renowned success coach.

What you believe to be true about yourself and your life runs the show. Your beliefs are on replay inside your brain like a recording playing over and over again. This source guides you to do or not to do things in your life.

I want to guide you to shift your priorities, so you can do the things that matter most to you. Let's take a deep dive and look at what means the most to you in your life.

Take out your journal and reply to the prompts below. Because everyone is different, this will help you to recognize what your beliefs are and what limitations you've created based on your beliefs, priorities, and life situation.

REFLECTION QUESTIONS

1. What do you prioritize in your life?
2. What can you RESTART with today?
3. What can you learn from your past behaviors?
4. What patterns of behavior are you willing to release?
5. What patterns of behavior contributed to your weight regain? What can you learn from this? What can you do differently to move you forward?

LIFE HACKS FOR DAILY BEHAVIOR CHANGE:

1. **Write down your plan. Keep it simple.**

   Keeping things simple will help you stay focused. Creating drastic change in a short time creates confusion, doubt, and overwhelm. Starting small and keeping things simple helps you to build behavior change over time. To create lasting change, maybe work on ONE habit change per week and track it from there. You will be able to recognize what improvements are being made and keep your habits, both sustainable and measurable.

2. **Identify triggers and replacement behaviors.**

   Your triggers are the emotions or situations that cause you to want to eat. Your replacement behaviors are the alternate behaviors that help you focus your attention on other activities rather than eating or food. Creating a list of activities that you can engage in will help you shift your attention away from food and help you stay busy and active.

3. **Focus on your replacement behaviors for at least 30 days.**

   Building consistency over time will ensure you're building new habits that focus on a lifestyle change.

YOUR 30-DAY DAILY ACTION CHALLENGE

For each day of the challenge, you'll either be thinking about the habit you want to change or taking action on it. The purpose of thinking about it is that you will be creating new thought patterns related to the behavior you desire to change. Try this series of 10-steps over the course of 30-days and see the change that occurs in your life.

1. Write down why it is important for you to change your behaviors and get clear on your desires.

2. Know your motivations. Your motivations are your deeper WHY and what you expect to gain from the outcome.

3. Establish your support system. Who will you call on when things get tough? Who will cheer you on, encourage you, and support you? Who will challenge you to keep going? Determine who they are now.

4. For every trigger you have, identify a positive replacement behavior that you can engage in instead.

5. Write down all the potential obstacles that could get in the way. Then write down all the ways you can overcome these obstacles.

6. Take ONE action every single day that moves you closer to your goals and desires.

7. Ask for help when you need it. Do not be shy or afraid to reach out. Use the team you established in Step 3.

8. Track your progress daily or weekly. Write down the good and the bad. Use awareness to help you learn, redirect, and grow.

9. Celebrate successes regularly. Looking back on your week could be a great way to see your successes and pump you up for growth.

10. Go back to step 1 if you are struggling, fall back into old habits, get lost or distracted, or find yourself discouraged in any way. Feeling free to start over is the key to success. No matter what goes on, you can always begin again.

CHAPTER 6

Reject the Perfectionistic ALL-or-NOTHING mentality

Perfectionism will keep you stuck ... period. And, here's a thought that will make you gasp—There is no such thing as perfect.

Yet so many within our community are gloriously committed to perfectionism. You are not alone here either. I am a recovering perfectionist myself. In fact, my last coach double-dared me to publish my last book before I had it edited for the third time, leading to crazy reviews about grammar. At first, I was mortified. I was dying inside. I was freaking out that I had let her push me outside of my perfectionistic comfort zone. And guess what? I didn't die! And you won't either.

And, you know what? I'm still alive. Since then, I've also realized that not being perfect makes me pretty cool. You know why?

I've done the inner work. I know I'm good enough. I know my worth. I know that what I'm doing is needed and valued. I also know that when other people cannot see past mistakes, however, they show up, they themselves are stuck in their own cycle of perfectionism, which is not about me, it's about them.

People will look for flaws in things when there is something in the messaging that makes them uncomfortable. Another psychologist's friend told me that when people have to critique you, it is because they can't deal with the truth in your message, so they must pick you apart to feel better about themselves and reduce their own cognitive dissonance. This is also akin to messaging from the famed psychiatrist Carl Jung: *"Everything that irritates us about others can lead us to an understanding of ourselves."*

Essentially, when we see things in others that bother us, it relates to an unhealed part of ourselves. As my psychologist colleague shared, we must resolve the discomfort that it creates. The perfectionist is always seeking to live up to either their own or others' perfectionistic ideals. There may be an extreme conflict that arises internally, which sometimes equates to someone or something else being "wrong" to justify their own "rightness." The perfectionist is always seeking to be perfect, even when this ideal is unrealistic. Instead of looking within, which could potentially be painful or cause discomfort, many look externally to find the inconsistencies and imperfections. This temporarily reduces one's discomfort and houses the blame elsewhere.

COGNITIVE DISSONANCE AND THE WLS JOURNEY

Cognitive dissonance is an inconsistency in one's thoughts, beliefs, attitudes, and behaviors—especially those related to behavioral decisions and attitude change. For example, when someone speaks about the required behavioral changes for post-op life, and they know what to do yet are still engaging in pre-op behaviors, they experience cognitive dissonance.

In other words, they know WHAT to do, and they aren't doing it.

Essentially, they have beliefs and behaviors that are conflicted or contradictory. This conflicting action and belief can create an uncomfortable feeling that leads to a need to resolve it—cognitive dissonance.

When you speak with someone about changing their behaviors, and they reply, "I know, I know," they are experiencing cognitive dissonance. They also want to minimize the discomfort of knowing. By bringing it up, they vocalize their knowledge, "I know, I know," because they want to change the topic. Their knowledge of the misalignment causes discomfort, and they are seeking to avoid feeling it. They know when something is not good for them, but they do it anyway. It's like someone who knows that smoking can cause cancer, yet they light up anyway.

When you start to speak the truth in a situation, and people dislike hearing about it, they will typically look for ways to diminish the truth you speak. Everyone experiences cognitive dissonance in different ways and throughout life, not only within the weight loss journey. The need to resolve the uncomfortable feeling can turn into rationalization or making excuses. This helps to reduce the uncomfortable feeling. It may show up as "it was just one cupcake," or "I don't know what came over me." In whatever way or form the resolution arrives, it is part of the cycle that many are caught up in because their beliefs, identity, and behaviors are not in alignment.

To reduce cognitive dissonance, you have a choice. You can change your beliefs, or you can change your behavior. Changing your behaviors is more challenging yet can help you the most. If you change your beliefs to "cake is good for me,"—it does not make the cake good for you. You've only changed your beliefs, not the result of the belief. Behavior change is an important part of your weight loss journey, and so is your identity. Who you are and what you believe is part of your identity; this can also impact what you do or don't do.

You can continue to rationalize, make excuses, and change the belief; or, you can take responsibility for the behavior, forgive yourself, create accountability, and change the behavior. Changing your behaviors is possible and doable. Starting one step at a time is doable. Taking on too much too soon is not.

Remember that wisdom is not the same as knowledge. You can know what to do, and still not do it. Wisdom is the application of knowledge.

THE SHAME SPIRAL & COGNITIVE DISSONANCE

Inside this process of reducing cognitive dissonance as you work to change your behavior, there will likely be critical. You may experience criticism from others or even from yourself. It's like that time when you dieted in your 20s, and your mother looked at you eating a cookie and asked, "Aren't you on a diet?" I don't know about you, but just hearing that example brings about feelings of shame, uncomfortable emotions, and feelings of cognitive dissonance (being out of alignment). Internal or external criticism can feel overwhelming, loud, and extremely disempowering. They saw you, and they called you on it. Ouch! We're talking about cognitive dissonance and criticism to help you understand it, so you can reduce the shame spiral that many individuals have experienced on their weight loss journey.

Brene Brown uses a quote in her book *Daring Greatly* that originated with Theodore Roosevelt, *"It is not the critic who counts; not the man who points out how the strong man stumbles, or where the doer of deeds could have done them better. The credit belongs to the man who is actually in the arena ..."*

This quote is about owning your strength, your willingness to try again, and again, despite criticism, despite the stumbles that you may experience on your journey. The critics' words are not what counts. It's your willingness to continue in spite of them. Acknowledge that you will fall down, and many will see you. Instead of feeling shame or sadness for having fallen, recognize that you only succeed by continuing to try and that the only failure is the result of quitting—not the result of trying.

The critics are loud. Whether the critics you experience are people in your life or the negative voice inside your own head, you can transcend them. You can overcome the past, and work through your own process with confidence, grace, encouragement, and love. Again, you will mess up. You will make poor choices at times, and it is up to you to learn from it— or not. It is up to you whether you choose to live by the old story and old dynamic or whether you step into the new habits, patterns, and new lifestyle.

I hope to guide each and every one of you, reading this to a place where you challenge yourself in an empowered, loving way. A place of self-acceptance and self-love even when you have to get real with yourself. Acknowledging that this journey is hard isn't shameful. It's recognizing that you are strong, and everything you are going through is meant to grow you and heal you. I hope to guide you to a place of striving for bettering yourself, regardless of the critics. It may be the inner critic who is shouting and screaming at you, and I hope to guide you to quiet this voice as well. I hope to guide you to a place where you can work on continually getting better and focus on improvement rather than your failures or what you did wrong. Continuing the cycle can be dangerous. Such perfectionism has been linked to disordered eating and body image issues. (Bardone-Cone, 2007). When the perfectionism cycle continues, the failure rates go up. This is because the intense pressure to succeed and fit into a box can, in fact, stop you from achieving anything. If you don't allow yourself to make any mistakes or gain knowledge from them, how do you expect to learn?

When you focus on your mistakes, you are engaging in perfectionistic thinking. When you shame, blame, or guilt yourself for "not being good enough" or for not creating consistent behavior change in two weeks' time, you are engaging in perfectionistic thinking. And it's not healthy. It's self-shaming, it's abusive, and it's awful.

You are not a machine. You are human. You are worthy, and you are loved, just as you are.

Here's the thing, on this journey, you will most definitely make mistakes. It's not a matter of IF, but a matter of WHEN. Everyone will make mistakes. This is part of being human. This is a part of the journey.

You will fall down. You will struggle. You will hit the wall a few times. If you don't, I'd be surprised. I would actually worry if you didn't make mistakes, missteps, and have struggles. It's all part of the process, and it is something all of us go through, and none of us are perfect. Instead of striving for perfection, why not go for excellence? Achieving is great. Perfectionism, however, is self-destructive and ends up setting you up for failure because it cannot be achieved by anyone. Once you get close to a goal, you likely move it because it wasn't "perfect enough" yet, and so the cycle begins. Let's look at the three types of perfectionists: other-oriented perfectionists, self-oriented perfectionists, and socially prescribed perfectionists (Silverman, 1999).

Self-oriented perfectionists turn their perfectionism inward on themselves. They typically set high standards for themselves in their careers and in regard to performance. They set high and unrealistic goals and self-standards. They focus on flaws and engage in self-criticism as a method of ensuring they achieve their goals.

Other-oriented perfectionists tend to be externally judging of others. They hold others to high standards and are highly critical of others and what others "should" be doing. They see all the ways others can improve, focusing their attention on what everyone else is doing wrong and how it can be improved.

Socially prescribed perfectionists are highly self-critical. The pressure they put on themselves to be the best is enormous. They worry they will be rejected by others. They also have very high expectations of themselves and how they should look. They focus on social norms of body image, how they are perceived by others, whether others will judge them, like them, hate them, and so on. These individuals focus their entire attention on how they are perceived by others and attempt to focus their lives on being perfect in the eyes of others. They have high perceived external standards, which leads to low-confidence, self-doubt, and anxiety.

Acknowledging that these patterns of perfectionism are dangerous can help you move beyond them. Don't forget that this process is about learning and growing. The expectations you may have for yourself are likely completely unrealistic. As a result of perfectionism, many individuals with maladaptive perfectionistic tendencies, such as rumination over past events, or a fixation on mistakes, often tend to engage in passive or avoidance coping. Rather than dealing with their problems or issues directly, they indirectly reduce emotional tension by eating, procrastinating, or engaging in other maladaptive behaviors. This both perpetuates the perfectionistic cycle and makes the problems that the person does not address even worse. Perfectionists often use intense self-criticism as a coping method, which makes them feel worse. All these patterns can also lead to cognitive dissonance when their behaviors and intentions are not in alignment.

Active coping, on the other hand, is a behavioral coping ability in which a person faces into their stress and deals with difficult situations or issues head-on.

This was failing and trying and struggling is all part of the journey. Instead of fearing it, expect it. Get ready for it. Prepare yourself and get excited for messing up, because when you do, you get to practice picking yourself back up again. (I will talk more on this in Chapter 9.) However, if you attempt to undermine it with perfectionistic tendencies, expect it to get worse.

For now, working on letting go of perfectionism is allowing yourself to create balance and do something even if it is only for five minutes.

5 WAYS TO LET GO OF PERFECTIONISM

1. **Start a movement/fitness routine for 10 minutes.**

   Walk outside. Walk on the treadmill. Go to the gym and ONLY stay 10 minutes. Allow yourself to do the absolute minimum. Your perfectionistic thinking will likely tell you it is not enough. Do it anyway.

2. **Allow yourself to finish short of perfect on a project.**

   Done is better than perfect. Then reflect on how it feels to be finished despite your typical expectations.

3. **Talk to yourself like you would a child you love.**

   When learning something new, you would not chastise a child for not "getting it" fast enough. You would likely be patient, kind, and loving. Use this encouraging, loving voice with yourself as well.

4. **Challenge yourself to look at risks vs. rewards, and then, of course, follow-through.**

   Many perfectionists become procrastinators because they fear not doing it right. What are the risks if you never start? What are the risks if you do mess up? What would the rewards be if you just got started? What would the rewards be if you started sooner rather than later?

5. **Try making a meal, and instead of freaking out, have fun with it.**

   Create a funny name for the recipe to get you started. Invite friends if it makes it easier. Make it playful, just like a child would. Expect to have messy counters. Expect that it might not turn out how you think it will. Instead, enjoy the process of getting through it and have fun playing with each step of the way.

REJECTING ALL-OR-NOTHING THINKING

Another way perfectionism shows up is in all-or-nothing thinking. Either you do everything perfectly or not at all. This is problematic because no one does everything awesome all the time. This is another reason to aim for 80/20 in all areas of life. Approximately 20-30% of the time, you won't be where you want to be, and that's okay.

However, if you end up criticizing or chastising yourself for those things, you'll be creating further emotional turmoil and stress. I bring this up because most often, my clients are their own worst critics. They end up being the one that creates the unrealistic principles that they cannot reach. The problem here isn't trying or reaching for excellence. It's that they shame themselves into a corner.

In a subsequent chapter, I'll share the importance of celebrating your successes on the journey, which helps with reducing the all-or-nothing thinking. Take time to recognize what 80% of a healthy lifestyle is for you. We often don't have an operational definition of what that is for us. We use other people's or society's general expectations and, again, that puts us in a box. It sets us up for failure because not only must we be perfect, but we also have to do it the way that "that guy" set it up.

This journey is yours, and you get to choose what works best for you to live a balanced life. That may mean meal planning twice a week instead of once a week. That may mean walking your dog daily rather than hitting the gym twice a week. The whole point is that you are moving in the direction of health and taking action daily toward where you want to be. Most people don't start off having it all figured out, and neither will you. That's why this is a process. Having to do it all today is super overwhelming. Breaking it down into smaller chunks makes it easier and doable.

Breaking the all-or-nothing begins with breaking things down and deciding what that looks like for your life. Aim for progress on your journey over perfection.

What progress can you make today, even if it's a tiny bit?

REFLECTION QUESTIONS

1. List at least one person you know who is perfect.
2. List out five things you can do today, imperfectly.
3. How might your perfectionism be related to people-pleasing? Do you have an innate desire to be praised?
4. What is the result of not being perfect, or not doing things "right"?
5. Which type of perfectionist are you, and how has this impacted your life?
6. How much do you value perfectionism in yourself and others? How harshly do you judge yourself and others for not being perfect?
7. In what other areas of your life might this be showing up?
8. What fears do you have about letting go of perfectionism?
9. What might happen if you let go of perfectionism and took action regardless of struggles, stumbles, and potential obstacles?
10. What does 'starting small to live a balanced life' look like for you?
11. In what ways do you fear starting small or starting at all?
12. What is the best thing that you could gain from starting small with one step today on your release your regain journey?
13. In what ways has the all-or-nothing perspective become a problem in your life?

14. How has all-or-nothing thinking kept you from getting things done on your WLS journey?
15. In what ways can you begin to start to engage in encouraging or empowering self-talk that helps reject perfectionism, and helps create incremental change?

CHAPTER 7

Reinforce Lifestyle Change

"And the day came when the risk to remain tight in a bud was more painful than the risk it took to blossom." – Anais Nin

Lifestyle change is totally different from the DIET mindset.

Diets are short-term. Diets are restrictive and punitive—diets end. Lifestyle change lasts forever. Lifestyle change is about creating balance. It's about living fluidly and flexibly. Lifestyle change accounts for indulgences, and honors balanced healthy living.

Lifestyle change is designed to help you commit to a series of behavioral changes over time. That is why it's forever. There's a different rhythm to it. For example, it's about doing the best you can day-to-day, giving yourself grace, then kicking it up a notch, and essentially, it's like a dance. Ever seen the cha-cha? Two steps forward and three steps back, then three steps forward and one step back. Its fluid, it's engaging, and it's consistent movement. Lifestyle change is about living flexibly versus trying to fit into a dress in six weeks.

So many people fall off track here. They focus on the short-term rather than the long-term. They focus on what they are missing out on rather than the life they will gain. They focus on foods they can't have, rather than what they can have and figure out how to make those delicious.

The diet mindset keeps people stuck in a loop, and it's not pretty!

The holidays are a time when people struggle with weight gain and regain. Because they haven't adopted lifestyle change, instead, they go back and forth with overeating and dieting. Instead of indulging once or twice and living by the 80/20 (healthy vs. unhealthy) principle, they go off their plan completely and end up feeling awful when they see they have regained weight.

Dieting is NOT a lifestyle. It's punitive.

Dieting is a cycle that perpetuates restriction and deprivation.

Diets are not meant to last. Diets are meant to be short-term.

Diets don't work when you try to live them forever.

And, if you try to live them forever, at some point, you reach a breaking point.

When you do, you end up sneaking food, hiding food, or even worse, binging. If you find yourself in a cycle of dieting and overeating, and cannot seem to get out, you may need to work with an eating disorders therapist to dig into the deeper issues that may be going on.

In contrast, lifestyle change is not punitive. It's not a punishment. It's not meant to be awful.

It's meant to help you live REALISTICALLY. It's a balance. It's flow.

Lifestyle change is about creating healthy habits. It's about changing your mindset around food and your behaviors. If you find yourself saying, "I can't have the small bag of pretzels on the plane," then you're likely on a diet.

Lifestyle change accounts for flexibility and fluidity in your plan. It's about thinking differently and accounting for the office party on Friday, or the monthly birthday celebrations, or those damn donuts that show up at the weekly meeting. DAMN THOSE DONUTS!!

You get to decide what is most important and what is least important to you. The food is always going to be there. It's not going anywhere. People will continue to bring food into work that isn't healthy. People will continue to celebrate with food. Your family will likely continue to bring food into your house that may not be on your plan.

This journey involves you adjusting your mindset to food, not banishing all Twinkies from the planet for eternity.

However, many individuals don't know how to adjust to lifestyle change because they have been so engaged in the diet mentality. The diet mentality becomes all they have ever known, so they cling to it. Because many perceive lifestyle change to be less restrictive and less like a diet, the expectation of immediate results causes people to engage in drastic measures. The diet cycle creates near-instant results on the scale. Although these results are short-term, many look for them to prove to themselves they can do it. However, the diet cycle is harmful and not sustainable for the long-term. Creating an 80/20 pattern with food, lifestyle habits, and behaviors are preferred to garner long-term results.

Now is the time to create your commitment to a lifestyle change. This begins by making a list of foods that you can make bari-friendly or "barify." Bari-friendly foods are foods that are higher in protein, lower in carbohydrates, and moderate in fat. These meals help you to eat moderately and sustainably. While many believe they can go back to eating the same foods they ate pre-op, they may experience weight regain. Opting to swap out a regular tortilla for a low-carb tortilla, for example, can be a great alternative, especially as a bariatric patient. Many other alternatives to pasta, bread, and other carb-laden foods are also available.

I've also met quite a few post-op patients that say, "Well, I'm not willing to do that," or "I'm not willing to give up that food." It's clear that this obstinance is part of their resistance to change or fears that emerge. When one approaches lifestyle change with inflexibility or obstinance, it will only affect that person's life and outcome, not anyone else.

Only you have the power to choose what you do and do not do. You have the power to choose the low-carb pasta alternative over the full-carb pasta. The choice is yours. However, if you encounter resistance to making these lifestyle changes, you may want to look deeper into what is going on emotionally. Most people that do not want to give something up to have a fear of loss or a fear of missing out. Some individuals gain all of their pleasure from food, and in their minds, losing this could cause even greater emotional pain. Each individual struggling with obstinance to behavior change must look into this for themselves. Finding alternatives is possible, but if you are obstinate that you will not change, then you also must be okay that nothing will change. As the saying goes, "If nothing changes, nothing changes."

Lasting lifestyle change occurs over time. It is not a light switch. It doesn't just happen. It's intentional, gradual, and requires a practice of new behaviors. Clients and others will often ask, "Where do I begin?"

Here are 6-steps to gradual behavior change to create lifestyle change:

Step 1: CLARITY. This first step is all about reflection and preparation. Focus on what you want to change and the outcome you want to create. Motivation comes from getting excited about the intended results and then taking action toward them. In this step, you will reflect on where you are stuck and look at the repeating patterns. The purpose here is to practice awareness to change the pattern. For example, if your issue is impulsive eating, you may need to practice mindfulness. If your issue is emotional eating, you may need to create a practice that allows you to check-in with your emotions and find alternative behaviors to soothe. If you are unaware, you will continue to spiral through confusion. This step gets you clear so you can decide what to work on.

Step 2: DECISION. Decide what action steps are needed. You must take a stand for yourself and decide to commit to a plan. It may not be about food. It may be about moving your body daily. It may be about water intake. Or, the plan may be about shifting your negative self-talk, or journaling. The point here is for you to decide. Often, I see others taking advice from professionals (psychotherapists, coaches, nutritionists, doctors, etc.) and not taking action. Then they feel bad or like failures. When you are fully invested in the decisions of your direction, you become fully invested in the process. While many fear being put in control of their own process, it is actually a cornerstone of success. It can be easy to sluff off others' recommendations, but when you commit to something that you created, you feel a deeper obligation to yourself. If you do not meal prepping, you may need to decide on what meals you will prep, how often you will do it, and how many steps you will break it down. You do not have to do it all at once. You get to break it down. You get to make it work for you. You get to be in charge of the process. When you follow how others do it, or how others recommend it be done, that may not work for you. Deciding on how you will eat healthily or move your body will create a greater commitment to your path and your process. Decide on your plan. Commit to a specific time when you will take action. Put it on your calendar like a doctor's appointment if you need to, to ensure you have it scheduled. Break things down into small chunks. Make it doable for your schedule. Again, your decision can be anything on your path. The most important thing is that you DECIDE to engage with ONE new behavior that you'll implement.

Step 3: FOLLOW THROUGH. This is the step where you walk the walk. This is the step where you take action on your decision. People often tell me, "This is where I get stuck; why can't I just follow through?" Here's the thing you must *want* to follow through. You have got to be excited about it. If you are not excited, go back to Step 1 or Step 2. You are creating the plan, so guess what? It gets to be exciting. It gets to be something that will change your life and something you are excited to take action on. Following through is not punishment. It is not something that someone else told you to do. It is the action you take after the commitment you made. Many people get stuck in, "I don't want to," and they rebel. If you are struggling with rebellion, go back, and recheck your readiness for change in Chapter 1. You can want something and be resistant to it at the same time. Sometimes it takes being angry and frustrated with where you are in order to propel you to where you want to be. You can change. You can commit. You can follow through.

Step 4: CYCLE. Consistency is the goal of any lifestyle change. It's the cycle that you are aiming to create. Repeating the same steps, day-in and day-out achieve results. What you do ONCE isn't what matters; what you do every single day gets you to the goal. Through the new behavior cycle, you'll learn great new habits. The first few times through, however, the new behaviors are not habits. They are still foreign until you have used them repeatedly. Keep going. You'll get there. Also, if you start to get bored, go back to Step 2, and find new ways to make your process fun, interesting, or exciting.

Step 5: LEARN. In this process, you will make missteps and mistakes. So, ask yourself what you can learn from this to grow. Maybe you need to shift the time of day you are engaging in the activity or break it down into even smaller chunks. Maybe you need to get an accountability buddy. Maybe there are emotional stressors that stand out. Whatever the challenge might be, see it as something you CAN and WILL overcome, rather than something which has conquered you. Additionally, go back to Step 2 and revise your plan once you've recognized what you've learned from this step.

Step 6: REPEAT. All the phases need to be repeated over time. This cycle requires frequent re-engagement and reentry. When creating habit change that will become a lifestyle change, it must be integrated into your life. Some of your other current habits might also change. This is a fluid process that requires flexibility, openness, and creativity. When you are creating this process for you and your life, it does not need to fit into a box. As I've said before, you get to create what fits and works for your life, and you can make it happen. It takes dedication and imagination to create the time and make it a priority in your life. You are worthy of a healthy, vibrant life, and you'll get it when you commit to the steps that lead you there.

Step 7: COMPASSION. Knowing when what you need is a swift kick in the butt due to your excuses, and when what you need is a break, kindness, and love is a fine line. Knowing the difference is key, so you don't end up beating yourself up for "not doing enough." Compassion is self-kindness. It is what you would say to your friend when they are struggling. It is the encouragement you would give to keep going when things get tough. It is also the tough love you might provide when becoming too lax or apathetic towards one's process. Being supportive and loving is important, whether you are struggling or achieving. Compassion, encouragement, and self-kindness are needed for both occasions.

REFLECTION QUESTIONS

1. What might lifestyle change look like for you in your life?
2. What fears come up for you regarding engaging in a lifestyle change?
3. Describe your perception of the difference in lifestyle change from dieting?
4. What resistance do you have toward creating lifestyle change?
5. How has the diet cycle shown up in your life?
6. What have your biggest issues from the diet cycle been? How has the diet cycle impacted your relationship with food?

7. What foods can you "barify" in order to help you create delicious menus of foods you enjoy?
8. What resistance do you have to change your behaviors?
9. What resistance do you have to food alternatives?
10. What resistance do you have to change your food choices?

CHAPTER 8

Relinquish Control

Right about now, all the control freaks are freaking out and trying to figure out how to completely avoid this chapter.

The cycle of deprivation and overeating is one example of a control cycle. Too much and not enough is part of that cycle of control. For those who struggle with eating, disorder control is one of the central themes. Those who struggle with anorexia exert too much control over abstaining from food—to their own detriment. Those who overeat may feel completely out of control with their food—to their own detriment. Those who binge also feel totally out of control and can't seem to get enough. Both ends of the spectrum shame themselves for how they look (body image) and their food choices. All have issues with control.

Punishment or reward centered around food is part of the problem, not the solution.

Creating a balance, a middle ground is essential for a long-term lifestyle change. And yet, those who struggle with sugar may say that they cannot have it in moderation. I totally understand. I am not one of those people, but I have many clients who have that issue, and sugar is a struggle for them. For this and many other reasons, I've partnered with a bariatric nutritionist who gives solid nutrition advice for those who struggle with sugar. No one size fits all. Knowing yourself and what you can and cannot handle, especially when sugar is involved, is the key.

While being in control of our choices is important, we also must let go of things outside of our control and not let food control us.

So often, I'll see people who want to control every aspect of life. This all-encompassing control is not possible. When we so desperately want to be in control, it could be a response to trauma—an attempt to feel safe and secure.

Uncertainty is everywhere, and getting comfortable with things being outside of your control will help you adjust to life's stressors.

If you are someone who has a history of trauma, you may need deeper work in this area. If you have a history with trauma, I highly advise that you seek out a therapist specializing in trauma. They will help you work through any deeper issues that may be present. Although the actions you've taken may not be healthy, your mind may have used them to keep you safe in one way or another. That trauma may have held you in a pattern of being and maybe keeping you from taking new action. Therapeutic work can help heal the trauma while allowing deeper work to facilitate you moving past it. A saying that is painfully true, "Your trauma was not your fault, but healing is your responsibility."

While the pain you experience from the past or the present is likely outside of your control, the only thing you have the ability to change is you. Even attempting to manage your healing process is a form of control. In order to heal, one must first recognize that they are in a cycle that needs to be healed. Control can be a part of this cycle. Recognizing this cycle can be very cathartic as well. Control as a pattern is rooted in fear. Surrender, on the other hand, is a path rooted in trust. While seeking to be in control can be a trauma response, that is not always the case. Learning about the cycle of control can be very empowering, and the good news is, patterns of control can be modified. They can also be very healing. Many can work through these patterns on their own. Learning to surrender is a skill to be learned for those struggling with control. It can also be very empowering to release the need to control everything.

Here's a little activity to get us started.

JOURNALING ACTIVITY

Take out a sheet of paper and draw a line down the middle. On one side, write down what is within your control. On the other side, write what is outside of your control. When you look at what you've written, first check that things outside of your control are truly outside of your control. For example, traffic jams are completely out of your control. But, leaving on time is within your control. Furthermore, the death of a loved one is out of your control. Getting grief therapy and eating healthy is within your control. I share these two examples with a purpose. I often see bariatric patients lose themselves in things they cannot control while minimizing or avoiding things that they do have the power to change. Gaining insight on how to better take care of yourself is instrumental to your growth, your emotional health, your physical health, and releasing your regain.

1. When you look at these two lists, what insight emerges regarding your perspective of what is within your control or outside of your control in your life?
2. What might be a new perspective you can adopt on taking back control over your behaviors?
3. What might be a new perspective you can adopt about releasing things outside of your control?
4. What fears do you have about being out of control?

5. How has overcontrol helped you in your life thus far?

6. How would you describe the control cycle in your life?

7. In what other areas of your life have you struggled with control, force, or cycling through the pattern of control vs. feeling out of control?

CONTROL AND AVOIDANCE

Another part of the control and out-of-control cycle can be avoidance. Not too long ago, a client came to me frustrated with her behaviors. She had been struggling with some emotions and admitted she didn't want to fully feel them out of fear they would send her into an emotional spiral. Instead, she emotionally ate, watched TV, helped others, and engaged in avoidance and distraction activities. We discussed this openly. She shared that she knew she was fully engaging in activities that continued the pattern of avoidance and weren't helping her to deal with what was coming up. We analyzed her patterns together and worked on coming to terms with the emotions she was avoiding. What came to light was a cycle of control.

She shared that she felt totally out of control when it came to her feelings, and as a result, she felt out of control with food and other behaviors. Conversely, in other areas of her life—at work, for example—she felt in complete control and able to function well. This success made her feel powerful and encouraged her pattern of trying to be in control. Her attempts to control her emotional state led her to feel out of control in other areas because they represented the fallacy of control. The fallacy of control is an internal locus of control where a person believes their success is based on an increase in perceived effort. Additionally, they believe there is a right way that things should be done. As a result of this pattern, they become frustrated if the results they receive are not the same as their expectations, despite the effort they put in. Additionally, this fallacy of control can show up in expectations to be perfectionistic, or as a caretaker. Both these roles typically believe that things should be done a certain way, which leaves them feeling disappointed and unfulfilled when they are unable to meet such standards.

Individuals relying on the control fallacy are typically working from an internal locus of control where they put themselves in control. They become frustrated, stressed, overwhelmed, angry, and resentful when they feel out of control because they are no longer in control of what they have created.

For my client, her pattern of trying to control everything actually led to many out of control behaviors, leaving her feeling frustrated and like a failure. We worked on her allowing things to be less than perfect while accepting a lack of control in certain situations.

As she worked on letting go of the need to be in control, she began to feel more empowered and less anxious over time. It was a process that included her being open to feeling her uncomfortable and unpredictable feelings and emotional states.

CONTROL VS. TRUST AND SURRENDER

Another pattern I often see within our community are those that stalk the scale. They weigh themselves fairly frequently and pay close attention to whether the scale goes down or up. They are committed to that scale and give so much meaning to the numbers that appear on it. The scale can also cause the cycle of control to get out of hand. At the beginning of this journey, when you first had surgery, you likely noticed the first bit of weight low in just a week or two. The speed of loss was related to the anesthesia and other factors associated with surgery and recovery. At your current stage, a few years or more after surgery, you've entered a new realm. Getting back on track and expecting to see instant results leads to pressured expectations. This can also lead to stress and fear-based thinking. Distorted eating can follow if you're not careful, which can also lead back to the diet mentality.

As you recommit to your journey and releasing regain, you also must commit to trust and surrender. The weight will likely come off slower. You'll likely have periods of stagnancy where the scale doesn't move. A multitude of reasons can cause this, and they differ for males and females. Regardless, you must trust that if you are doing what you need to do behaviorally, you will see a shift. It may just take a little longer.

Patience is required. If you become impatient because the scale isn't moving, you will likely get very frustrated and angry with yourself or your plan. You'll likely try to do ten different things (maybe even dieting) to try to shift the scale. This cycle of impatience is all part of the problem. Using all the insights in this book, I am confident you can release your regain. However, if you push yourself and your body, giving it the equivalent of an ultimatum, I will also promise you that you'll likely see an even longer stall.

You can compare it to watching and waiting for water to boil. The emotional tension is high, and you become aggravated and exasperated by your lack of results. But it's not that you won't have results, it's that you must trust and surrender to your plan. When you are eating healthy, moving your body, and working on your mindset, it will come off. When you have committed to the basics and begin to live fully, you will see it come off. However, the push that happens with impatience often creates an internal conflict that leads you to do something rash or extreme. Releasing your regain isn't about doing something extreme; it's creating a healthy lifestyle you can live with for the long-term. This is important to remember. You want it, and you want it now. I get it. I truly do. And, your impatience may actually cause more harm than good when you distrust your body and the process itself.

At this point, I often see people flip-flop from plan to plan, expecting different results. When they don't get it, they end up even more frustrated, and then they end up returning to no plan. When on no plan, they unfortunately regain. In chapter 2, I shared why I get frustrated with those who plan-hop. It's because I know it doesn't work. It's not the *plan* that works or doesn't work—it's your ability to stick with ONE thing long-term that matters the most. Whether it's a balanced macros plan, keto, AIP protocol, gluten-free, or low-carb—it doesn't matter. Each individual must choose the best plan for themselves. The point is to stick with what you choose and to stop plan-hopping with the latest fads. That's dieting. That is NOT lifestyle change. For a small portion of people with specific medical conditions, it may make a distinct difference. Sticking with ANY plan long-term is the most important part, and that's where the mindset piece must be applied. For most, the plan doesn't matter as much as sticking with it. Without the correct mindset, many end up back in the diet mentality, which often leads them back to suffering and frustration.

The amount of control is not what helps you to lose weight. It is the trust you have in yourself, your body, and the process that helps you to lose weight. Forcing your body to lose in your time frame causes more stress, not less stress. Allowing your body to lose weight in its time is a process of trust and surrender. When you are taking action and following the plan, your body will lose. Sure, some minor adjustments might be needed, yet all in all, trust that your body is adjusting is key. "Know thyself" can also be applied here. If someone does not know the patterns of their own body, they may be struggling to trust the changes that are happening. They may be more inclined to take drastic short-term measures to see immediate changes. However, short-term measures do not produce long-term results. This reality is essential to remember when the desire is to acquire lasting change.

REFLECTION QUESTIONS

1. In what areas of your life do you feel out of control? In what ways does this show up?
2. In what areas of your life do you feel the need to control? In what ways does this show up?
3. Have you ever diet-hopped, and if so, what did you learn from it? How has it helped or hurt your weight loss process?
4. In what ways have you been patient and impatient with your weight loss process?
5. What is your typical pattern when you reach a weight-loss stall?
6. In what areas of your life do patterns of mistrust or distrust of yourself or others appear?

7. In what areas of your life would it be most important for you to build trust with yourself?
8. What might happen if you decided to let go and trust yourself, your body, and the process?
9. How can you apply trusting yourself, surrendering to the process, and releasing control to your weight loss journey?
10. What fears do you have about releasing control?
11. What fears do you have about trusting yourself and/or your body?

CHAPTER 9

Redirect Mistakes

Ahh ... mistakes. This area is where I see a lot of people get stuck and fall all over themselves.

Mistakes, missteps, and poor choices happen. They are not the end unless you choose for them to be. You can choose to beat yourself up, shame yourself into oblivion, or even quit. But this doesn't work. Instead, it makes you feel worse, and you are more likely to overeat. Mistakes are part of the process. Accepting this is necessary to losing weight and keeping it off.

Like I said in earlier chapters, you can RESTART and RECOMMIT at any time.

It's very common for people to make mistakes, to make poor choices, and to feel bad about it.

None of us are perfect, and we are not expected to follow the guidelines 100% of the time, because perfection is not possible for anyone.

So often, we think that holding ourselves accountable is the same as holding ourselves to a perfectionistic standard. It is not. If you are a perfectionist, we are going to work on you, giving this up and letting this go. We've talked about part of this in a previous chapter, but this chapter is all about embracing mistakes and learning from them.

Mistakes are always teaching you and guiding you. Wisdom is in each and every mess-up, poor choice, wrong move, hiccup, etc. Insert grace, accept the decision made, and seek to gain as much as you can from it.

As I've said before, at least a zillion times, this process is a lifestyle change. It's not a diet. If you find yourself downing a handful of chocolate-covered raisins without a thought to only subsequently berate yourself because you forgot you were trying or "lost your head," then it's time to take a step back and reevaluate. It's time to look at the reason that happened. It's time to put a process in place that helps you to pause between urges, triggers, and eating.

Mistakes don't hold you back from greatness, the self-punishment and internal downward spiral created from your own self-talk keep you stuck. Shame begets more shame. Shame begets more eating off track. Shame, blame, and guilt only creates more negativity that leads you to self-soothing with food.

There will be angst. There will be frustration. You are absolutely allowed to feel that range of emotions. Instead of beating yourself up, use that anger and frustration to get up and get better. Keep trying. Keep going. Continue to challenge yourself and learn from these mistakes because mistakes don't go away. They don't stop—ever. They are part of the process. They are scattered around on the road to success.

Instead of thinking, mistakes are blocking you ***from*** success, begin to see them as lessons on the road **TO** success. They exist to teach you about yourself, your emotions, and what may be going on within you.

One of my favorite sayings on this journey is, "It's not IF you mess up, but WHEN you mess up," because you will. Not because I have any doubts about you, but because we will ALL fall on the path at times.

I'm here to tell you that I mess up all the time. However, I've maintained my weight loss because I use the mistakes as fuel to drive me to my better self. I learn from it, and I move on.

I have learned that beating myself up is like playing for the other team. If I want to win, achieve, and succeed, I must be willing to be the best I can be on my own team, for my team, and my team is ME. To do this, I have to learn to dust myself off, pick myself up, forgive, learn, and keep moving.

I use the example of Olympic athletes all the time because even they mess up. Sometimes the athlete favored to win the gold ends up falling on the ice during the semi-finals; it happens. And, they get back up and start again. They keep going despite the challenges.

So how do you do it?

Start by paying attention and talking to yourself. You've got to be aware of what is going on, when it typically happens, and take note of it so that you can insert a pause in that space next time. The pause gives you the opportunity to choose differently.

NEUROPLASTICITY & THE ABILITY TO REDIRECT MISTAKES

An amazing amount of psychological and brain research has been done in the area of neuroplasticity. Neuroplasticity, or brain plasticity as it is sometimes referred to, is essentially the ability of the brain to modify and re-wire connections, creating new neural networks. This ability allows us to continue learning throughout our lifespan and is one of the foundations of new habit formation. When you are changing your habits, you rely on neuroplasticity, or the creation of new neural networks, in order to reorganize your thought patterns into what you want your new habit of being like. A brain is a powerful tool, and it can do almost anything you put your mind to.

When we focus, using heightened awareness and practice, we have the power to change how we think and behave via neuroplasticity.

The way I explain it to my clients is this: Imagine that you have a set of neuropathways that run like a superhighway in your brain. This superhighway is comfortable to drive on because it's the route you've always taken. Maybe along this superhighway, you've developed habits you want to extinguish. Along this highway, you may have conditioned yourself to graze on snacks after 9 pm, eat emotionally for comfort, and have a pattern of avoiding all physical activity.

Using neuroplasticity, you can rewire and reprogram your mind. As a result, you also have the tools to think and behave differently. Our brains are the master computer. Once we have mastered training our brains, we have the ability to change all things in our life. When you focus on rewiring your brain, you can literally accomplish anything. The brain is the master tool that you control in order to be, do, or have anything you desire. Once you are in control of your brain, all the other systems fall into place.

CHANGE YOUR BRAIN: STEPS TO CHANGE USING NEUROPLASTICITY

1. **Embrace challenges (rather than avoiding them).**

   When you embrace challenges, you take on opportunities to grow with new experiences. You are required to consciously think, plan, and carry out the necessary steps of the challenge, which helps you to build new neurons and new neuropathways. This helps to advance your skillset and give you a sense of accomplishment.

2. **Take on new experiences.**

Taking on new experiences, in general, will help expand your mindset and expand neuroplasticity. Each new experience prompts a change in one's brain structure, function, or, potentially, both.

3. **Engage in activities you enjoy or find fun—or learn to see the fun in them.**

Triggering neuroplasticity with new activities doesn't necessarily mean they will stay. Engaging in fun activities triggers your brain to repeat behaviors that are enjoyable and challenging, encouraging you to practice these again and again. It is through practice that neuroplasticity creates lasting effects.

4. **Seek out peak experiences.**

Peak experiences is a term coined by Abraham Maslow in 1964. These experiences are described as rare, exciting, stimulating, wonderous, and a moment accompanied by a euphoric mental state. These experiences are moments of happiness and fulfillment when someone is in an optimal state. These peak experiences are triggered by varying activating events that are different for everyone. They typically have characteristics that include elements of significance, fulfillment, and spirituality. The significance of the person may lead to greater awareness and understanding that serves as a turning point for the person.

Fulfillment in peak experiences generates positive emotions and is internally rewarding. Spirituality is represented as a feeling of oneness with the world, and individuals may experience a sense of losing track of time while participating in the peak experience.

5. **Keep using important skills regularly.**

Using important skills regularly helps to continue building neuroplasticity and developing the brain through continued practice. You can practice these skills and implement them in a variety of ways. It could be the expansion and practice of cognitive skills using memory and using challenging brain activities or of kinesthetic skills such as learning a new dance or how to play a new instrument. Learning a new language, changing how you exercise, including how you move your body (practicing Zumba, yoga, or swim aerobics, for example) and playing games regularly are all ways to practice important skills and consistently practice developing neuroplasticity. The more the activities are practiced, the more developed the neuropathways become.

6. **Visualize or watch anything you want to do better.**

Visualization is a great way to rewire your brain with neuroplasticity. Many athletes use visualization to improve their performance on the field. This impacts neuroplasticity as your brain cannot distinguish the difference between real and imaginary. Therefore, using visualizations of you engaging in a variety of experiences can help prime your brain to take appropriate action in that activity. Visualization also helps promote empowerment and increase in motivation to engage in the desired activity. Positive self-beliefs and new neuropathways are built just by visualizing yourself engaged in new activities. Visualization is easy, too. Close your eyes, and picture yourself as if you are watching a movie on a big screen. Watch yourself engaging in a behavior that promotes healthy living. Be sure to infuse engaging in this experience with positive feelings. Notice how this experience alters your reality in your body. Most people share they feel a sense of calm and accomplishment just by engaging in visualization. (A full step-by-step guide to conducting visualization is included in Chapter 7 of *Bariatric Mindset Success*.)

EXPERIENCING RELAPSE & REDIRECTING MISSTEPS/MISTAKES

If you have read any of my other books, attended one of my lectures, or joined one of my online groups, you know that I'm not a food addict. You also know that I don't talk a lot about food addiction. It's not that I don't believe in it. Some individuals are hard-wired for food addiction or sugar addiction. Personally, I am not one of those people, and most of the people who follow my work aren't food addicts either. They are emotional eaters and recognize themselves as such.

Many professionals in the field discuss food addiction and work with people on it. I specifically address emotional eating. My work focuses on retraining your brain and reprogramming your mindset to believe in yourself and overcome polarized thinking.

As many people talk about mistakes and missteps, I wanted to include the topic of relapse from a different perspective—from an emotional eating perspective and from a behavioral perspective. In Chapter 1, I discussed the transtheoretical model of change, also referred to as the stages of change. Within this model, a section refers to "relapse" or falling back into old behavioral patterns. This is true for any behaviors and not exclusively for patterns of addiction.

When you fall back into old patterns, this is a relapse—moving backward rather than continuing on the path forward.

When a relapse occurs, I believe individuals go back to a previous way of doing things. They fall BACK into old habits. Even the model, stages of change, includes the possibility that a person may be doing well with continued action towards maintenance and still may struggle with a period of relapse.

When you relapse to emotional eating, it is largely because you've let an old habit back in, or you've gotten too comfortable with specific behavior.

In my practice, I often see individuals who have relapsed after a period of intense stress, such as experiencing grief and/or loss of a loved one or a life-altering change like a move cross country or a job loss. Any number of things can trigger a relapse. In my experience, though, when I've seen individuals struggling, they've lost their ability to cope with daily life due to extreme stress, leading them to pause any progress on their journey. This break may lead to a setback that then leads to increased feelings of failure, which can lead to isolation and engaging in self-destructive behaviors out of frustration, fear, hopelessness, and learned helplessness. It's also an opportunity, however, to shift gears and take back your power. Many things can be done to redirect yourself and learn from mistakes along the way. Asking for help, reaching out, and connecting with a support network can create a greater sense of belonging while helping someone recognize they are not alone and what they are experiencing is normal.

Everyone has setbacks. Everyone has issues on the journey. The fear of reaching out is a normal fear, and it is the one that often leads to regaining. When people fear they might be judged based on their perceived failures, they are less likely to reach out for help. However, reaching out for help is the one thing that will most likely urge them to return to their plan, re-engage their process, and start to see success. Unfortunately, fear often wins. Reaching out for help despite the fear is essential for your growth. In this community, we all recognize how difficult this journey is. It's time to reconnect, recommit, and re-engage with your process in order to recover from relapse.

FROM RELAPSE TO RECOVERY

With recovery, you can forgive yourself for the struggle. You can forgive yourself for whatever choices were made at the time you made them, and you can pick yourself up and choose again. You get a do-over. You get to learn from the experience. You get to refocus your attention on what you want, rather than beating yourself up for what you did not do.

The process of rebuilding yourself and experiencing recovery is acknowledging that the temptations are there. It is acknowledging that you aren't perfect, you will slip up, and you'll intentionally catch yourself and pick yourself up when you do. Recovery also involves acknowledging your own triggers, and a recommitment to your journey. This whole process is about embracing the learning from setbacks in order to set yourself up for a comeback.

Furthermore, emotional eating is a very complex issue with many facets. Getting to the underlying cause can be a process in itself for most people. Being able to name your feelings, examine your feelings, and gain a deeper understanding of how you feel is essential. Being able to name your triggers, examine your struggles, and acknowledge them for what they are is all part of the process. Digging into your past, your childhood, trauma that you may have experienced, or other emotional issues along the way may be required. You may need them to surface so that you can deal with them. Working with a therapist to heal the trauma and the emotional pain while guiding you back to yourself may all be a part of this process.

Allow yourself this process. Allow yourself to heal. Emotional eating is not about food. It does not happen because the food is so good you cannot help yourself. No. Emotional eating is about emotions. It is NEVER about the food.

CHAPTER 10

Rejoice in Mini successes

As discussed in previous chapters, it is not the BIG overtures that determine your results, but the small steps over time.

Everyone wants a restart that seems to put them through the wringer. This is not necessary.

You need a series of small steps over time that will create a lifestyle change. Yet, for your brain to be stimulated, you feel you must start something BIG.

Through your mini successes, you can create a big change in your life. However, many of the clients that I have worked with through the years don't seem to see these small successes as significant.

They think they "should" be doing them and that they don't count. So, they minimize their successes.

In my group coaching program, I always start by asking my participants what their successes have been for the previous week or two. The purpose of this is so they can write down and share aloud what they have been doing RIGHT.

So often, bariatric patients ONLY see what they are not doing yet, what they are doing wrong, and where they aren't yet on their journey.

If you only focus on where you are NOT, you'll only see what you are not doing, rather than the steps you ARE taking.

This is why successes are important to track.

One of my regular clients is famous on our group calls for frequently coming on, saying she has ZERO successes to share. So, I'll make her go through her week step by step, telling me what she HAS done for herself.

Inevitably, she will find 3-5 things that she has been doing well that are considered successes. After doing this over and over, she has grown tremendously in her self-belief and in knowing she has successes even when she thinks she doesn't.

When we lead with a negative mindset, we focus our attention on what we are doing WRONG rather than what we are doing right, and this becomes part of our programming.

This programming is part of the thinking that leads us to feel defeated about ourselves when, in reality, it is all perception.

I have my participants ALWAYS start off with their successes so they can fully embrace their efforts and what they are doing well.

How might you need to embrace your own successes? Or do you have a habit of focusing on what you haven't mastered yet? Or are you focused on all the mistakes and missteps you've made in the last week or so? What is your focus, success, or failure?

Try writing down your successes at the end of the day:

- What have you done today that would be considered a success?
- Did you avoid celebratory food in the break room?
- Did you get in all your water?
- Did you go for a walk on your lunch hour?
- Did you track all your food?

- Did you set boundaries with a toxic family member?
- What did you do today that could be labeled a success?

Start looking for things that you ARE doing right and build on them daily. Then keep up the consistency with looking for what you are doing right. You will always find laundry lists of things you are doing wrong.

Reminder: NONE OF US ARE PERFECT.

The goal here is to improve your state of being, and if your focus is on all the things you've done wrong, you'll end up feeling even worse. Then, if your pattern is like many others when you feel worse, you eat.

Let's break the cycle.

It's time to learn from the mistakes and grow from them. No one succeeds by "scarlet lettering" themselves. No one succeeds by replaying all the things they have done wrong.

Instead, examine the evidence, look for the growth opportunity, and move on. Then practice this way of thinking again and again. This practice and celebrating what you are doing right will give you the encouragement to keep going and reach your goal weight.

When you shame yourself for all the things you are not yet doing, you end up creating more self-hatred and self-loathing that really does not need to be there.

It may seem normal and natural to look at what's wrong, yet very few people look at things from the perspective of what is going right. This happens especially when people focus on the scale as a singular measurement of achievement. The scale isn't always a good measurement of behavior change. You may have eaten balanced and healthy all week, exercised, drank your water, and taken supplements and still no movement on the scale.

Behavior change must be rewarded for itself, and not dependent upon the scale for achievement's sake. The scale will move. If things are going right and you're living 80/20, the scale will move. This is the point in which you must trust the process and not skip out on the daily action steps.

The mini successes are in the day-to-day. The mini-successes are the mini-breakthroughs that you've been working on for so long. The mini successes are the celebration of your new habits and the times you remembered, the times you took action, and the times you redirected yourself when you were struggling or had urges or temptations.

ACTIVITY: START TRACKING YOUR DAILY SUCCESSES

No matter how small you think it may be, take out a sheet of paper or your notebook that you've dedicated to this process and write the date and "Today's Successes" at the top of the page.

Think of at least 2-3 things you have achieved today that contribute to your journey or activities that contribute to where you want to be.

It can be as simple as drinking 64oz of water or going on a 10-minute walk. It can be that you tracked your food intake in your *Bariatric Mindset 3-month Accountability Workbook* or in an online app. It could be that you stayed on track with your food today and did not graze. It could be that you avoided the donuts in the breakroom today and drank water instead. It could be that you called a friend when you were really upset about getting passed up for a promotion instead of eating your feelings.

You likely have many successes on a daily basis that you fail to recognize only because you are not looking for them. Today is the day we begin looking for them, seeing them, and celebrating them as part of your new mindset routine.

Try this daily for a week and notice how your perspective changes about your process.

REFLECTION QUESTIONS
1. What successes have you achieved along your journey?
2. Which successes are you most proud of?
3. While there may be plenty of back to basics successes, what successes have you noticed in how you feel about yourself, or in your body image?
4. What non-scale victories can you celebrate weekly or monthly?

CHAPTER 11

Release Negativity & the Past
(Relationships, Commitments,
Boundaries, Jobs, etc.)

You may have heard this before, the life you have is a result of your thoughts, beliefs, and emotions about what's available to you. What you THINK is available to you is what you end up receiving. What you think about most is where your brain most often goes. What you focus on expands.

"When you change the way you think about things, the things you think about change." – Wayne Dyer.

I've used this quote often in the work that I do on purpose. It is because we have to shift the way we see things in order to create change within our behaviors. (Hey perfectionists, I'm repeating myself so that you will see the patterns here and recognize how everything is connected.)

When you release negative or disempowered thinking, you essentially break the chains of those thoughts and beliefs. When you choose a different thought process, you empower yourself, and in turn, you change your outcome and your life.

Who you always were, will not determine who you will become in the future. You have the ability to change your story, to change the script, and to create a new ending for yourself in your life. Although many bariatric patients may have had a history of trauma, that does not mean you have to continue to carry that with you into your future.

SEXUAL ABUSE, TRAUMA, OBESITY, AND REGAIN

Many professionals agree that obesity is difficult to treat because the causes are complex and not completely understood. While the focus of many programs is largely on food and exercise, many forget that there can be psychological underpinnings that affect obesity treatments. One of the major psychological issues for individuals struggling with obesity is a history of sexual abuse or sexual trauma. Research shows childhood sexual abuse survivors are significantly more likely to become obese than non-abused individuals. Another interesting report is that those who have been a victim of sexual abuse have been shown to be relatively treatment-resistant in terms of their obesity.

In my own practice, I've noticed individuals losing and regaining weight after weight loss surgery and not understanding why. After uncovering a history of sexual abuse, it becomes evident for many that feeling unsafe in their new thinner bodies becomes a key factor in their weight regain.

Most frequently, I will hear clients tell me about how they feel unsafe in their thinner bodies and uncomfortable receiving attention. They preferred to be invisible yet fight to be thin. It can present a frustrating dynamic, especially when one's focus is to reach a healthy weight. These psychological factors can present a difficult pattern that causes individuals to feel something is wrong with them. Unhealed trauma can stay within the psyche and the body, creating patterns of behavior that will leave you stuck within a vicious cycle – not knowing how to stop it or exit the cycle for good.

Therefore, this factor must be addressed within our community. Food and exercise alone cannot contend with or solve some issues. Obesity can be a defense mechanism. Dealing with the emotional trauma that lingers from past sexual abuse needs to be dealt with in counseling for individuals to recognize that other patterns may be contributing to their obesity. The weight loss and weight gain cycle can be largely due to a complex string of emotions that include worthiness, safety, security, and seeking protection.

For those reading this, if you had not dealt with past sexual abuse, regardless of when it occurred across your lifespan, it is strongly urged that you seek counseling to work on these issues in therapy. Untreated sexual trauma may continue to perpetuate obesity. You are not alone and can work through this with qualified and trained professionals. Sexual abuse is not a topic to work on in coaching but should be handled very specifically with a licensed counselor who is specially trained in helping people with sexual trauma.

I can provide all the tools, journaling prompts, or activities in the world to help people shift their mindset and their patterns, but if they have not dealt with unhealed trauma, the patterns leading back to regain will emerge again at some point. I highly recommend those with these issues, which may be coaching with me, to also work with a skilled therapist to address the trauma. When releasing your past, many may forget the trauma that has gone untreated, or unhealed. Treating and healing your trauma is central to your overall healing and a key to losing regain, shifting the lose/gain cycle, and creating lasting weight loss.

RELEASING THE PAST

Many people have gone through divorces, losing loved ones, job loss, and so much more. These life situations and stressors, while awful, are not a reason for you to stop living. They are also not reasons for you to quit or put your health and wellness goals on hold. I frequently see individuals putting themselves on the back burner to deal with life issues, and as a result, they have regained. Lifestyle change can help here because it is a complement to dealing with life struggles. It's not an add-on experience that you bypass because you have to press pause. The lifestyle changes that are recommended in this book are meant to help you get through the struggles. They are meant to help guide you through to a healthier you, even when it feels like life is throwing lemons at your head.

You may have temporary setbacks on your weight loss journey, and it may take a while for you to gain your bearings again. This is another reason to work on the mindset piece of this lifestyle. Many clients that I have worked with have told me that they would be in a much worse place had they not committed to the mindset work. Because of the mindset work they did, they didn't return to food to soothe. The practices they cultivated and behavior change that they created led them to continued self-care when they experienced struggles in their life.

No one is immune from life struggles or tragedy. Everyone has an opportunity to behave differently, to cope differently, and to work through difficult times once they have new knowledge, a new mindset, and new practices they can implement if and when life gets tough. This process is about helping you to create a new pattern of beliefs, a new set of behavioral practices, and lifestyle change that supports the life you desire to create.

Once again, here's a recommendation for those who may have experienced any type of trauma in the past to work through such issues in a counseling environment. Through the coaching that I conduct, I strongly suggest that clients with a history of trauma see a therapist while they go through my coaching group. The therapy is fundamental to their growth. The coaching is a great compliment to their therapy work to move them farther and faster once they have dealt with the deeper issues that have held them back.

The old thoughts may be that you "can't" or that it's too "hard." Essentially by repeating these to yourself over and over again, you're continuing to reinforce that same pattern that you "can't" or that it's too "hard." So, that becomes the pattern continued within your mind and your lifestyle. It is the pattern that can become the psychological condition termed "learned helplessness."

The term *learned helplessness* was originally coined by Dr. Martin Seligman, who is also known as the father of positive psychology. He discusses this term in-depth in his book, *Learned Optimism*. The condition of learned helplessness is a generally defined belief that one is incapable of accomplishing tasks or goals as a result of little or no control over their environment. This is also the person that has the "why bother" mentality, and who subsequently gives upon themselves. It can be the product of trauma or repeated exposure to aversive stimuli. Over time, when people are unable to achieve their goals, they inevitably stop trying or give in to perceived failure—they experience learned helplessness. This condition causes individuals to overlook opportunities and conditions for change. Learned helplessness can also be associated with several different psychological disorders such as depression, anxiety, and phobias. All of these conditions can be exacerbated by learned helplessness as well.

Here are some steps to lead you to overcome learned helplessness:

1. **Recognize and accept this new awareness and get to the root of the pattern.**

   All learned helplessness starts somewhere. Whether it was rooted in childhood or in repeated patterns of behavior, you'll likely look back on your life to find a common denominator that has impacted your path and who you are today. Write this down or record it somewhere so you can begin to unravel the pattern and the limiting beliefs that are intertwined in your pattern of learned helplessness.

2. **Identify your limiting beliefs.**

   When you have limiting beliefs, they play like a program of what you can or cannot do. When you can identify how your thinking is limited by these beliefs, you can change them.

3. **Reframe limiting beliefs.**

   Reframing one's beliefs is a technique used in therapy to help create a new way of looking at a situation, person, or relationship by changing the meaning of the thought. Also referred to as cognitive reframing, this strategy is often used in therapy to help clients look at situations from a slightly different perspective. Start by writing down the limiting belief. The reframe itself should analyze the limiting belief. Is it true? Or is it false? Is it subjective or objective? Also, think of the emotions and feelings that the belief brings up in you. Write down any other thoughts about the belief. Then create four alternative thoughts and list evidence to support the alternative thoughts. Write down the feeling or emotions experienced with this new thought and belief.

4. **Be mindful of your self-talk.**

How do you talk to yourself and about yourself? Change the negative self-talk into positive self-talk. In order to change the pattern of learned helplessness, the pattern of self-talk must also change. You need to recognize and record the automatic self-talk that reinforces the old negative beliefs, and then rewrite the self-talk to be more loving, supportive, and positive.

5. **Practice the new positive self-talk over time.**

Don't just recite or use the new self-talk once. It's something that is to be cultivated and practiced over time. The process of catching yourself and changing the dialogue/monologue inside your head can be pivotal to shifting the self-talk and decreasing the pattern of learned helplessness.

6. **Improve self-awareness through journaling or personal reflection.**

One of the things I tell my clients frequently is that they don't have a filter inside their head to filter out the negative talk. We all have a sensor that stops us from saying vile, hateful things to others, but no such censor or filter inside our own heads protects *us* from these things. Journaling is a fabulous tool for writing out new awareness, patterns, thoughts, feelings, and situations that bring up difficult emotions, uncomfortable emotions, or self-criticism that may surface over time. In this way, journaling can help reduce learned helplessness as a record of shifting how you talk to yourself and analyzing the negative and shifting it to a more positive monologue inside your head.

7. **Set small goals that require you to take daily action.**

   Goals are great; however, people often create goals that are large and way out of reach. Setting small goals or weekly goals with daily action tasks can help you change your habits. These small steps can also give you immediate proof that you can make changes and achieve results in a short time.

8. **Change your environment to help you achieve your goals.**

   People frequently make decisions based on environmental cues, and this can leave them feeling frustrated if they fall into old habits. If you consistently see cookies on the counter, they may need to be housed in a cabinet instead. If you are frequently triggered by passing Dunkin' Donuts on your way to work, maybe taking a different route for a while will help you break the habit. If visiting your sister's house triggers you because of all the candy jars she has, ask her to come to your space instead. These are just a few examples of how your environment can impact your behavior and what you can do to change it. Changing your environment in a way that supports your goals can help with behavior cues and reduce habituated thoughts and desires. New environmental cues can be set up to support your goals and establish a new space that could cultivate a positive outcome.

9. **Celebrate small wins.**

Celebrating your successes reinforces the attitude that you can achieve what you've set out to achieve. It also helps unravel the pattern of learned helplessness because the successes will become compounded over time giving proof to the new pattern of behavior.

10. **Look for the silver lining in difficult situations.**

What might this situation or experience be teaching you? How might it be elevating you beyond your current situation? The silver lining may be the lesson learned, or an opportunity to strengthen something within you. Instead of seeing it as something awful, how might this situation or experience be changing you to help you become stronger, better, or move you farther along in your journey?

USING MINDSET SKILLS FOR GROWTH

Another development in mindset research in recent years has been the two mindsets that shape our lives. Dr. Carol Dweck of Stanford University wrote about them in her book, *Mindset: The New Psychology of Success*. She states that individuals are likely to come from two categories, growth mindset or a fixed mindset. In her book, she states that a "fixed mindset" assumes that character, intelligence, and creative ability are static and unchangeable. These individuals see failure as final or fatal and believe that intelligence is static and necessary for success. According to Dweck, an individual with a "growth mindset," however, thrives on change, sees failure as part of the process, and recognizes that intelligence is fluid and can come in a variety of forms. Individuals with a growth mindset are more likely to learn from mistakes rather than seeing mistakes as detrimental.

A growth mindset is integral for one's post-op journey, especially in releasing regain because this entire weight loss process is fluid with ups and downs, gains, and losses. If someone is to attach the meaning of failure or giving up to anyone step, they have essentially committed to the end, when in fact, it may just be a temporary obstacle. This journey has a variety of twists and turns with next to nothing being static or stagnant.

In order to move into this new way of thinking and being, you must be open to changing the way you have always thought in order to get to new ways of being and acting.

Another phrase is often used to describe old patterns that people become committed to, "Old ways won't open new doors."

Dr. Dweck's book has been revolutionary in the fields of education and success coaching. However, it has rarely been used in the field of weight loss or bariatrics. I want to introduce some of the principles for developing a growth mindset as developed from Dr. Dweck's work and apply them to our community of bariatric patients. Learning how to develop a growth mindset would be a great asset to our community and change the way we learn, grow, lose weight, and maintain weight.

Here are 11 ways bariatric patients can work to develop a growth mindset in their post-operative journey towards a lifestyle change. A growth mindset changes the neuroplasticity of the brain and helps individuals become more adaptable and resilient to change, helping individuals challenge their abilities and become more dedicated to practicing in order to cultivate success.

1. Acknowledge and embrace imperfections.

In order to embrace change, one must acknowledge their weaknesses in order to work on them and overcome them. This is growth.

2. **View challenges as opportunities.**

This teaches individuals how to fail well. This also reminds me of Michael Jordan sharing how many shots he missed rather than how many he achieved. Failure is part of growth, and opportunities to grow are found in challenges.

3. **Try different learning strategies and tactics.**

Not everyone learns in the same way. Even among my private clients, I will have one client that succeeds using a particular tool, while another person, who might be trying to achieve the same goal, needs a totally different tool or strategy based on their personality or needs. Instead of giving up, try new tools and seek out new strategies to help you achieve your goals.

4. **Recognize your brain isn't fixed.**

You are always growing and learning. Imagine you've gotten a new job. You'll need to train yourself to drive to the new place of employment even though your brain may be attached to driving to your old office complex. Your brain will learn the new route with time and practice. Most other things in your life follow the same pattern— brain plasticity and neurodevelopment rely on practice and creating new neuropathways to support the new behavior you're trying to create.

5. **Remove the word "failing" from your vocabulary and replace it with the word "learning."**

No one is a failure in this process. You are learning new tools, new behaviors, and new strategies. Shift how you talk to yourself and acknowledge this is a process.

6. **Choose to value the process over perfection or the intended outcome.**

   Yes, everyone is trying to achieve a goal. Yes, everyone wants to release their regain and get to maintenance. However, if you don't enjoy the process and become present with the process, you'll likely start to judge the process and get frustrated with it. It's not the time it takes to get "there," but how you adjust to the learning curve that makes the biggest difference.

7. **Create regular opportunities for reflection on your process.**

   Those who reflect on their growth and behaviors do better than those who don't reflect at all. Reflection also helps in celebrating the good and recognizing what might need to change from day-to-day and week-to-week. It creates additional opportunities for growth, rather than criticism or judgment.

8. **Brain training and lifestyle change are synonymous.**

   This whole process is about retraining your brain to build new neuropathways so that you are creating and supporting healthy habits. The brain is a muscle that needs to be worked out, just like the body. Practicing this helps you to be more resilient and flexible.

9. **Cultivate grit.**

   Determination and perseverance are part of the process. Those who are able to get back up after being knocked down have been shown to have greater long-term success rates because they see the fall as temporary and an obstacle to be overcome rather than a flaw or self-fulfilling prophecy.

10. Be realistic about time and effort.

People often expect to master topics quickly and efficiently. Again, brain training is similar to training your body. You wouldn't expect to be a bodybuilder overnight, so don't expect to change your patterns or behaviors overnight, either. The same is true for weight loss. Attempting to master too much too soon can leave you feeling frustrated. Recognize that there is a pace to this process, and you can only master so much at once. Be patient with the process and see it as a process to be mastered. Once you do, you'll see the fruits of your labor. You will see the weight come off. It's through this process, and through your practice of these efforts over time, that you'll gain traction. Be patient. Be mindful. Take consistent action. Continue to put forth the effort.

11. Own your growth mindset attitude.

In developing a growth mindset, it is important that you acknowledge your emotions and your attitude and use them to help you to continue to master life challenges. If your attitude is negative or limiting, you may have reverted to a fixed mindset. A growth mindset sees all obstacles as part of growth and seeks to overcome those obstacles by embracing opportunities for continued learning.

CHAPTER 12

Review & Revise as Needed

No plan is perfect from the start. Having the ability to recognize what's working and what is not can help you achieve more in the long-term. You are not the one that may not be working. It could be that your plan needs revising.

However, rather than review and revise, many people judge themselves, give up or completely start over. Starting over is fine, except many will look at that last "plan" or "diet" they used as something that "failed." Please remember you are not on a diet; you are working to create a lasting lifestyle change. Remember that everyone will get off track at times because that is life. No one is on plan 100% of the time. Thinking they can be leads to all-or-nothing thinking. Instead, practicing the 80/20 ratio helps many create a plan with flexibility.

Let me be clear, again, the "diet" or "plan" you have used is not as important as how diligently you have applied it. The feeling of not having achieved results; however, can leave you feeling frustrated and like a failure. Mindset and habit changes are the goals now, not whether the "plan" has worked or not. This may sound harsh, yet it's true; no plan is going to work if you aren't going to actively work on it. Because of this, they are going deeper regarding the emotional resistance to change may be helpful for those who are really struggling with creating change in their life. The habits and patterns of the old lifestyle can be difficult to shift. This saying I love sums this up well, *"There's nothing wrong with you. You are just committed to a pattern of behaviors and habits that are no longer serving you."*

It's time to let these go. Revise your plan.

Through the realization of the patterns that are no longer serving you, you can let them go. You may grieve them. You may need to mourn them. And, in order to grow, you've got to release them. You may notice the resistance that wells up within you. You may feel yourself saying, "I don't want to," or "I'm not ready." This, my friends, is resistance. Go back to the behavior change model we discussed in Chapter 1 and look at where you may fall in those stages of change. Change always begins with you. It may be uncomfortable to grow, and yet it can be more painful to stay the same, in a place where you no longer belong.

Often after weight loss surgery, I see the grief that happens as people mourn the loss of their relationship with food. Some people grieve the loss of eating to soothe. People may still use food to soothe, and their grief may come later when they choose themselves, their healing, and their health over food.

The fear, the anger, and the frustration that comes up are likely linked to grief over the resulting need to change one's relationship with food. It may also be linked to the weight regain itself, especially if too much time had passed between when you stopped practicing lifestyle change and when you begin again. An internal struggle may be occurring. You may feel resistant to or rebellious about changing your ways. In whatever way this shows up for you, pay attention to it, because it is meant to teach you.

The patterns that emerge when you start to take your power back from food may give you even more insight and guidance to heal.

Notice I didn't mention any recommended dieting. That's because once again, what I'm talking about is NOT a diet. I'm proposing practicing behavior change over time. Our goals aren't about celery or carrots or tuna ... bleck! This process isn't about eating foods you hate, nor is it about indulging in foods either. We want to create balance and use new tools that create long-term habits.

As I've shared in earlier chapters, your plan may need revisions and redirections. The redirections aren't major overtures of switching from one extreme plan to another. Instead, they involve making changes to your day-to-day life that provide you with more structure or more guidance to help you along the way.

Many individuals are resistant to a structure. They want to fly by the seat of their pants. They want to do things when they "feel" like it. However, if you wait until you feel like doing something, you could be waiting a very long time. Discipline and structure are needed here.

Reviewing and revising your plan is necessary on a consistent basis. People get into ruts. They get into a certain routine that is comfortable but may not be getting the results.

Michael, 56, started a plan to lose his regain. He ate oatmeal every morning and visited the gym three days a week. He had a fairly typical routine, but when he noticed that he wasn't losing any longer, he started to panic. He thought he had to change things up significantly and did not know where to start. First, he started tracking his water. This helped for a short time, and he saw some weight loss—then he hit another stall. In this type of situation, reviewing and revising is necessary to implement new changes. Starting with one thing at a time can help guide things along. After review, he realized he was already eating fairly healthy and balanced, and he did not need to start a restrictive diet or change his food plan up significantly. Instead, he added an additional day of fitness per week and changed his gym time to two days of cardio fitness and two days of strength training. This new schedule helped him gain muscle mass and change his body over the course of the next six weeks. He also began losing again and reported feeling better.

While this may be a model story, Michael had to address other things that weren't included in the above synopsis. Michael had to work through feeling like a failure to reach a long stall in his weight loss journey. He had to resist the urge to restrict his diet significantly or to overeat when he felt awful about himself. Michael also had to think healthier about himself and his journey, which meant being patient with himself and his body as he implemented change.

Six weeks is a long time to wait to see change. It doesn't always take six weeks, but when it comes to seeing fitness changes, it can take that long to see it physically. People commonly become impatient and resistant. People want to try twenty different new things in an attempt to make the scale move. This can cause trouble because while our bodies are amazing, they are not machines. Many people have the expectation that a new plan means that they should see results immediately. However, plans don't always work like that, and reviewing and revising one's plan may also require planning and patience.

Getting impatient with your progress can also lead to perceived failure or even weight regain. Trying twenty different things and then getting frustrated that nothing works is a broader issue. It's impossible to know what step, strategy or technique works if one is throwing everything they have at the wall. Slow and steady is a far more successful strategy than attempting to do everything all at once.

ACTIVITY: REVIEW & REVISE

Step 1: Take a deeper look at your current meal plan. Assess all aspects of your plan, including your food consumption, when you eat, how much you eat, and even write down your mealtimes. This helps you to evaluate whether you are eating too much or not enough.

Step 2: Calculate your water intake. Are you getting enough water daily? Or do you need more?

Step 3: Assess your fitness routine. What fitness, exercise, or movement are you currently practicing.

Step 4: Assess your current stress levels and mood. Do you feel stressed frequently? Have you implemented a stress management plan? Are any emotional stressors impacting your ability to implement your plan, or do you frequently experience stress, anxiety, or low mood?

Step 5: Assess your current sleep patterns. Sleep could be a reason your weight has stalled. If you are not frequently sleeping 5-6 hours or more per night, you might need a referral to your doctor for a sleep study. Problematic sleep patterns have been linked to weight gain and stalled weight loss.

From this overall assessment, choose ONE thing to focus on and improve in the next 6-8 weeks. One person may find integrating meal planning and preparation into their life is important. Another might find tracking as an integral part of their revision while yet another person might recognize that their stress levels need to be addressed and make mood management their focus.

Implementation of these more personalized revisions requires a clear plan. If you're not getting enough sleep, you might consider going to bed earlier or crafting a sleep hygiene routine. Obtaining an accountability partner and reporting in on progress and setbacks may be the key for others. Remember that setbacks are part of progress and should not be seen as failures. The growth dance includes some steps backward. Expect that you may fall back into old patterns. Use these backward steps as an opportunity to continue to shift and move forward beyond this behavior. Behavior change does not happen overnight. The process requires building consistency with the new behavior over time. People often forget the new behavior. Be patient and kind to yourself. Forge ahead and recognize that with each step you take, you are moving toward consistent change. The new behavior will take root. Continue to practice it over and over, and you will get there.

REFLECTION QUESTIONS

1. What is your pattern when it comes to reviewing or revising your plan?
2. What are your expectations when it comes to behavior change and seeing results?

3. How has your weight loss journey been impacted by your inability to be patient with the process?
4. What issues have come up as a result of impatience?
5. What have you learned about yourself, your process, or being impatient that could help you change your behavior and create a bigger impact on your weight loss journey?
6. What have you learned that may help you be more present and patient in releasing your regain?
7. What practices have you been using that you need to review because they may or may not be serving you the best on your weight loss journey?
8. What practices might you revise in your weight loss journey to help you achieve greater results?

CHAPTER 13

Recreate/Reinvent yourself

I get it. You don't really know who you are. I see it all the time.

Who are you, really?

You spend 24/7 in your body, yet you don't know much about him or her, do you?

I often see people who are going through the motions, day in, day out. Do you think you're actually living right now?

Get up.

Eat.

Go to work.

Come home.

Make dinner.

Eat.

Evening Routine.

Sleep.

Get up.

Eat.

Go to work.

Come home.

Make Dinner.

Eat.

Evening Routine.

Sleep.

Get off the merry go round, and live!

What do you do with your spare time?

Is that what you want to be doing?

Is your day job what you desire to be doing with your life?

Do you have any other passions?

Do you have any idea what you REALLY TRULY want?

Or are you afraid of digging into your dreams?

Ahhh ... there's the scary part. Actually, choosing what it is that you WANT to be, WANT to do ... WHO you would actually become.

This is a deeper issue, indeed. CHOOSING. DECIDING. COMMITTING.

You likely think you have to wait until you've lost the weight to figure that out. You don't. But you want to wait. You think you have to lose the weight to figure it out, and instead, it is the other way around.

In order to fully lose the weight, you have to take a stand for something, and that something is YOU. You have to know what you desire so you can go after it. You need to know what you want so that the motivation of your desire will give you a kickstart. From there, you'll develop the determination, the drive, and the discipline to keep going long after the initial motivation wanes.

If you don't fully embrace who you want to be, you'll likely continue to go through the cycle until you get fed up and quit.

This is the BEGINNING of your visioning process.

This is YOUR opportunity to dream about what you truly desire. But, will you allow yourself to go there?

People often feel unworthy of their true desires or even embarrassed to share what they desire. They are afraid they are silly or foolish. Dreams are neither.

So often, people will say "why bother" because of their own fear of not achieving what they truly desire OR because they are so deep into their unhappiness that they cannot even imagine what they could achieve or experience that would make them happy.

Others say "why bother" because they are mentally stuck in their current circumstances and cannot see any other options available to them. The difficulties they see can feel like roadblocks, and yet the only block is within their own mind. Einstein has been quoted as saying, "*We cannot solve our problems with the same thinking we used to create them.*" This suggests that we create problems within our minds, and changing requires giving attention to new and creative solutions. We can change the outcome with new solutions, as long as we become open to changing how we think in order to get there.

In my book *Bariatric Mindset Success*, I talk about finding your WHY. When you dig deeper into WHY you want to achieve success, this helps lead you to a greater understanding of your desires, your needs, and the WHOLE reason you want to work for it. This process is very similar. Knowing your WHY, creating a vision for your future, is fundamental to your process.

Often in my practice, there will be a client who says, "I'm too old to have a WHY," or "There is nothing that I want." Having no desire at all can lead some to use food as a stimulus because it can be exciting for the brain. It's a change. It's a thrill. Not having other things in your life that excite you can lead to using food for excitement, which leads you back to where you do not want to go.

Using food as the most exciting stimulus in life is also a way for people to stay safe and not challenge themselves to grow beyond where they are. The individuals most in this category are women in their 60s, 70s, and 80s—yes, 80s! They see their life as "coming to an end," and I'm consistently encouraging them to LIVE life to the fullest. It's not over, friends, you have more life left in you.

It's not how many years you have left in your life, but the life left in your years! I strongly encourage people to keep dreaming and keep doing for themselves. This keeps us invested in and excited about life.

Even as I was conducting my research for my doctoral dissertation, many of my research participants shared they had made a career change after having weight loss surgery. They shared that they felt overlooked and undervalued at work prior to their surgery. After their surgery, a majority of them shared that they felt so confident that they started to pursue their dreams. Dreams they had long forgotten because they had given up hope these dreams could be achieved while living with extreme obesity. This surgery is a second chance to dream and take action on what is desired to create in one's life. This process offers a chance of living fully.

No matter what they are, everyone still has dreams left in them. It doesn't have to be a career or a job—maybe it's a trip you'd like to take, or a place you'd like to see, or a thing you'd like to do. It is possible to achieve one's dreams, no matter what they are.

I've had clients tell me that they have traveled the world because they felt free to do so after losing the weight. I've had clients share that they've moved into a tiny house because that excited them. One client started a non-profit in her 60s because she felt passionate about a specific mission and was now fully able to run it after losing all her weight.

Life is what you make of it. Whatever the circumstances you are in, you can make a change. The limitations you perceive are all in your mind.

I've had clients go through horrible divorces and difficult breakups because, for so long, they were held emotionally captive by narcissistic partners, or partners they held on to because they did not believe they could or would find anyone else. I've seen clients move mountains for themselves in the most difficult of conditions because they believed in themselves. I've worked with individuals who have overcome trauma, abuse, and neglect to change their beliefs and their lives so they could fully step into the life they desired for themselves. I've seen clients come off of disability and create a new life for themselves. Whatever you desire, you can achieve it!

You may say, "Listen, you don't know me or my situation," and you're right, I don't. What I do know is that it doesn't matter your education, how much money you make or don't make, where you live, what your relationship or job situation is … if you want to make a change, you can and you will.

If you have a dream inside you, you can achieve it. It begins with your mindset and movement toward change.

Change begins with a vision. It takes a vision of something greater, something bigger, something that will spark joy in your heart and life into your soul.

Essentially, in order to recreate or reinvent yourself, you must first allow yourself to dream. Then, you have to open yourself up to believing those dreams can come true. Third, you must be bold and courageous enough to start taking action in that direction.

Absolutely everyone has the ability to change their life. You do not have to have any special talents or abilities. You must only have a belief in yourself and the belief in your dreams. This belief is where it all begins. The steps can and will unfold once you have committed to something you desire to achieve. Let's dig into what your big dreams are so you can recreate yourself and reinvent yourself.

REFLECTION QUESTIONS

What is the vision you have for the rest of your life?

What would you like to create in your life beyond the weight loss?

Who would you become if life had no limits?

How might you live your life differently if you sought to live a life beyond your perceived limitations? How would you want to feel? What daily or weekly activities would help you to feel that way?

What would you do with your life if there were no limitations?

What would you seek to create in your home life, in your career, in your relationships, or in other areas of your life?

What big changes would you make in your life?

What is the big dream you have for yourself?

What is currently holding you back?

What would you do if this wasn't holding you back?

What can you do to see this as an opportunity rather than an obstacle?

What can you do differently that would allow you to push through this situation and create the life you desire?

What would you do to make a difference in your life?

Would you travel? Would you give back to your community? Would you go back and get another degree? Would you seek advancement at work? Would you change jobs? Would you start a new career altogether?

Would you get back into dating? Would you improve the relationship you currently have?

Would you get involved in a hobby?

Would you volunteer or do something that gives back to others?

What would you do to fulfill your dreams?

THE "F" WORD

Finding fulfillment is one of the key ingredients to living successfully. Setting healthy boundaries will also help you to continue to take care of you as you seek this fulfillment.

We worked a lot of what you really want in an earlier chapter. This chapter helps bridge the gap between what you want and who you want to be. You may want a lot of things in your life, and yet you haven't figured it out yet.

Fear may be part of this for many reasons.

Fear may hold you back from achieving greater fulfillment in life. Judgment or criticism could hold you back, or fear of trying something new. You could also have a fear of failure or a fear of success. Many are afraid of success because of what it might mean. People fear success because of the new expectations that may be put on them if they do achieve great things. As a result of the fear of success, people may stop trying. Similarly, people fear failure because of the meaning that they would create in their lives. Actual failure registers differently for people than never taking the chance. As a result of this fear of failure, people may stop trying.

Fulfillment, however, has been the key to success for many, leading them to live fuller richer lives and creating moments, memories, events, experiences, and situations that they would not have otherwise engaged in prior to their weight loss surgery. Creating fulfillment has also been one of the ways many of my clients have achieved weight loss maintenance. They have found a greater purpose in living life that isn't focused around food but instead focused on experiencing happiness, joy, passion, and excitement in their life.

REFLECTION QUESTIONS

1. In what areas of your life are you bored or feel things are stale or stagnant?
2. In what areas of your life do you find yourself procrastinating, avoiding, or reaching for food because you're not happy or fulfilled?
3. In what areas of your life would you like to recreate or reinvent yourself?
4. What would be some ways you could change things up in these areas of your life to create greater joy?
5. Define what fulfillment means to you.
6. What activities, events, or experiences would be fulfilling for you?

7. What obstacles do you see to reaching or seeking fulfillment in your life?

8. How can you see these obstacles differently? What perspective shift might you need to change your thinking or perception of these obstacles?

9. What activities do you find fulfilling, exciting, joyous, or fun? What activities create happiness in your life?

10. Who do you surround yourself with who creates happiness, fulfillment, passion, joy, or fun?

11. What would you like to create that would help you to attain fulfillment?

12. What fears do you have around creating fulfillment in your life?

13. What fears of failure or fears of success come up when you think of living a life that brings you joy, passion, excitement, or happiness?

CHAPTER 14

Reestablish/Reintegrate, the Maintenance Phase

Maintenance is where everyone is heading and where everyone wants to be. Believe me! I hear people talking about getting to goal ALL the time. The thing is, if you don't know what you'll do when you get to maintenance, or ***how***-to live-in maintenance, you won't stay there long.

Living in maintenance is very different from being in the weight loss phase of your program. Maintenance requires creating a rhythm in your life. New structures, new routines, and new patterns must be created to carry you through your life. Successful weight loss maintainers are just as careful, concerned, and focused as those in the weight loss phase.

Successful maintainers continue to track their food intake. In the clinical literature, this is called self-monitoring. Individuals who have long-term success also continue to move their bodies regularly. For them, it's not about weight loss. It's about being healthy and feeling good. Individuals who track their food for the long-term using tracking tools such as My Fitness Pal, or other tracking or self-monitoring tools are doing so to hold themselves accountable (Burke, Wang, & Sevick, 2011; Butryn, Phelan, Hill, & Wing, 2007; Hartmann-Boyce, Boylan, Jebb, & Aveyard, 2018).

For them, tracking is an awareness tool, not a diet tool. They continue to use these methods to keep themselves accountable for their choices and to ensure they are staying within a certain range. They continue to walk the walk even though they are not trying to lose any more weight. This is because they aren't *dieting*. They are simply living wisely, living healthy, and continuing to create or make space for balanced living.

Maintainers make self-care a priority. They continue the patterns they learned in the weight loss phase and implement a new version of them for the next phase.

These individuals also know that lifestyle change is not an all or nothing pattern. It's a daily life pattern. If they miss one day, they make it up the next. They start over from the moment they realized they missed the opportunity, or they start over the next day. They aren't beating themselves up, crying about failures or missed opportunities. They pick up right where they left off, and they keep going. This mindset shift is needed to lose regain, and to keep it off. Successful maintainers recognize the balance in life and know that self-care isn't a luxury; it's a necessary standard of care. They recognize that in order to stay where they are, they must prioritize themselves.

If you walked into a hospital and they said, "Oh sorry, we can't give you a bed, that's a luxury," you'd likely get pretty upset. Beds are a standard of care. When you think about taking care of yourself, you're likely modeling what you saw your parents or caregivers model for you. People-pleasing doesn't help anyone but the person taking advantage of it.

You can be a helper, a friend, and a good person and still say no.

Saying no doesn't make you awful. It makes you human. It shows integrity. It shows courage. It shows self-respect.

You also have the ability to say yes. Using discernment about when to say yes, and when to say no is a learned skill. This discernment helps to establish new patterns for you and helps you remember that, just because someone needs something, it doesn't mean you must oblige.

Doing for yourself doesn't make you selfish, just like doing for others doesn't make you selfless. Like any other area, a delicate balance of love and respect is required for yourself and for others.

One night I was speaking at a support group meeting I visit a few times a year. The topic on this specific night was about setting healthy boundaries. I happened to be discussing the topic of self-care and saying no to others' needs as a form of self-care. A woman was eager to share and ask questions. I could tell she did not like my suggestion that people say no to other's needs or requests. She shared part of her experience and explained that she likes to help others because it makes her feel good. She started to get defensive when sharing. She shared it was such a huge part of her life that she didn't believe in saying no.

I asked her permission to ask a few questions about her patterns. She agreed. I asked her if during any of the occasions that she had said yes to help others if she had she felt regret, or resentment for saying yes because of exhaustion, overwhelm, taking on too much, or due to a lack of appreciation. She replied that she had, but immediately began to explain her way through her answer.

This was a key indication that she wasn't ready to stop people-pleasing. It was part of her identity. I wholeheartedly believe her when she said she loved helping people. I truly believe she does. However, she does it to her own detriment, and like anything, that is where the problems arise.

When someone extends themselves to their own detriment and denies themselves self-care for the sake of martyrdom, it becomes a bigger issue. People-pleasing comes up because people don't feel worthy to say no. They feel obligated to everyone else for one reason or another. Feeling wanted and needed fills a void. For many individuals who have struggled with obesity for any length of time, the need to please others is part of their own need to feel acceptance.

This woman had reached a goal and later shared that without food, she didn't know who she was anymore. She had not made the connection between her pleasing behavior and her patterns with food. Rather, her comment about not knowing who she was anymore was related to wanting to find her identity through helping. She stated that helping people gave her purpose and because she felt she had been given a second chance, she wanted to do the same for others. As she had already hit her goal weight, she struggled with her identity. She shifted away from food toward helping others as her focus, and she became out of balance in another area of her life.

The purpose of sharing this story is this: Maintenance is not only about weight and maintaining weight loss. It's also about maintaining a healthy balance in *all* areas of your life.

However, areas can pop-up behaviorally or emotionally that may have nothing to do with food. Other patterns of behavior, such as people-pleasing or approval seeking, can cause people to sacrifice themselves or lack self-care, which can cause issues in maintenance.

People-pleasing can lead to resentment and feelings of powerlessness that then can lead to overeating. I see many post-ops go through this cycle, and yet they don't even realize how their day-to-day behaviors are impacting their eating behaviors.

"Using food to soothe" is an overused and oversimplified phrase that doesn't show the battles that people face on a day-to-day basis.

It's used to describe the single mom who doesn't know how to stand her ground with her child's father on where to meet to change custody.

It's used to describe the woman who feels powerless in asking for a raise while seeing everyone else get promoted around her.

It's used to describe the man who hasn't yet come out to his parents and fears he'll be shunned.

It's used to describe the individuals who are eating in order to avoid feeling hurt, heartbreak, shame, angst, fear, anxiety, and a range of other emotions.

Most issues aren't food issues. They are unresolved emotional issues. Through these unresolved emotional issues and fears of rejection, people go above and beyond to be accepted in whatever way they can. Over and over, I see this in my practice. It's sad and frustrating for the individuals that are hurting and eating in order to cope and soothe these emotional issues. The food doesn't make the problems go away. Only through working through these emotional issues can they be resolved. In these cases, therapeutic interventions are recommended treatment.

Learning to deal with your emotions and all the things that go on in life will help you handle the food.

Some post-op patients may go from using food to soothe, to shopping heavily. Or from using food to cope, to using fitness or workouts to cope. This process isn't about moving from one thing to another, but instead creating a healthy balance across all areas of one's life. No life is ever completely balanced, but it's a good practice to seek.

If the emotions go unresolved or aren't dealt with, a host of other issues will inevitably surface, including regain. Throughout this book, I've focused on emotional explanations rather than advice like "eat 2oz of chicken." The food is just the symptom of a greater issue. Avoiding cupcakes will only get you so far because the cupcakes aren't the source issue.

I could write a nutrition book about chicken, beef, and veggies, but this is part of the problem I often see even in the weight loss industry. If you do not address what's underneath your food issues, you could read two hundred books on what to eat and still struggle with food. While people may struggle with what to eat, typically, they are actually feeling out of control with food, which is the emotional issue causing the problem. The struggles with WHY you are eating are more likely to lead to regaining over time than WHAT you are eating. Furthermore, the weight regain is typically not what you're eating, but what issues, problems, or stressors are taking place in your life. The rollercoaster in their emotional state, and thus in their habits, continually leads people to eat outside the 80/20 ratio.

An integration must take place in the post-op process here. Integrating healthy habits across all areas of life is vital to success. Creating a healthy balance in your emotional state and allowing that to infiltrate your habits and practices.

Many like to begin this integration process by focusing on the food. I see people all the time talking about food, what to eat, when to eat, etc. Once again, this will only get you so far. Yes, you will need to know what to eat and how to eat, but focusing on the food alone is a distraction. It's through the emotional shifts that you'll gain the greatest traction. It's through healing the emotional wounds that you'll be set free from food.

Again, food will be there forever. We all will continue to eat. However, when emotionally healthy, the foods you crave and desire will change because your view of yourself will change. You'll see food as something to nourish your body and something to be savored. When your view of yourself is hatred, disdain, or anger, you'll seek out foods to stuff down the feelings as fast as you can, to fill a void that you don't know how to fill any other way.

Maintenance after reaching one's weight loss goals is a bigger and broader topic. It's about living in fulfillment and joy. It's about creating a sense of balance using the 80/20 plan with food. It's about seeking enjoyment in other areas of life (outside of food). It's about seeking new challenges and growing outside one's comfort zone. It's about living your life to the fullest, regardless of your age or any other status. It's about not putting up with crap anymore and taking a stand for what you believe in, even if no one else does.

The maintenance phase is not only getting to your goal weight, but it's also learning how to handle tumultuous times with grace and flow. It is being prepared to live with and deal with life issues as they arise. I tell my clients that this whole process, including the maintenance phase, is like driving a car. You always have your hands on the steering wheel. When you take your hands off, you may veer to the left or to the right. You start to veer off the road, and if you veer too far, you could end up in a ditch. Similarly, when you keep your hands on the wheel, you are intentional, focused, and stay in the middle of the road. Also, like driving a car, however, you develop patterns in this new lifestyle that help you to create new healthy autopilot mechanisms as well. Just as anyone has likely experienced getting in the car and driving somewhere without thinking about it, the path does get easier. Initially, developing new habits is something you must consciously think about. Over time, like driving a car, you'll get more comfortable with the process, and it gets easier to do it though, this does not mean that you won't ever have issues. We all do. Everyone is bound to have difficult times in life. When you have mastered your relationship with food, the maintenance phase has been reached, and so has success.

Maintenance is not only about weight loss maintenance. It's about maintaining all of YOU—mind, body, and spirit. The thing many get stuck on, though, is the weight. They think the weight loss will solve everything, only to realize the rest of their problems are still there. Often, it's not the weight loss that people seek as much as it is the feeling or experience; they believe they will get once they get to their goal weight.

Gaining insight into what the maintenance phase might be like for you is important. You likely have a deep yearning to get there, but do you know what life will be like once you do? Do you have dreams that your problems will go away once you get to that goal weight, or that the food issues will have subsided?

Starting to project what the maintenance phase will be like for you will help you significantly because it can help you prepare for this phase in advance. Many individuals have a naïve belief that once they get to a goal, everything is peachy. Getting to the goal is one phase; maintaining that goal weight is a whole new animal.

The point in sharing this is not to be negative, but to help you to be realistic and once again share that this is not a diet. Once individuals hit maintenance, they stay, thereby continuing the daily practices that helped get them there. This lifestyle includes all the basics that helped guide you on this journey in the beginning. What helps people to be successful in the long-term, and keep the weight off beyond reaching the goal, is the lifestyle mindset.

So many parts of this journey impact your life that isn't about food or fitness. Much of this journey revolves around all the other difficulties, challenges, and struggles that impact your ability to follow any food or fitness plan. Once you work on your mindset, it becomes easier to face and overcome those challenges. This is how you can release your regain and maintain your weight loss.

REFLECTION QUESTIONS

I've created a list of journaling prompts for you to use as you go through this process. Some of these journaling prompts have multiple questions on purpose. Often, people are so incredibly excited to get to maintenance, and then, once they get there, it's a huge letdown. They typically don't know what to do next. Part of changing your mindset is beginning to envision yourself at maintenance and what that future you would do. How would you live? How would you eat? How would you move your body?

By starting to think about these things, you can start to create this vision in your mind's eye and plan for it. When people never think about getting there, they may end up realizing they weren't ready to be there. The goal is to get you off the diet cycle and into a long-term lifestyle change. This begins with the suggestions in this book, guiding you through your own visualizations and your own journey of what your life will look like. That journey begins with you. Use these prompts to expand on your own journey and to build an understanding of who you want to be, what you want to do once you get to a goal, and how you plan to live your healthy life in the maintenance phase.

1. As you look forward to maintenance with your weight loss process, what do you hope to experience in other areas of your life?
2. What do you expect maintenance to look like for you? Physically? Mentally? Emotionally? With your relationship with food?
3. What are your biggest fears about maintenance?
4. What excites you the most about getting to goal and maintaining your weight?

5. How is maintenance different from the weight loss phase for you?

6. What do you expect to achieve once you get to maintenance?

7. What emotions or feelings do you hope to have in maintenance? What can you start to "feel" on your way to maintenance even if you haven't hit your goals yet?

8. What would it be like to hit your goals and to maintain your weight and life at that goal? How would that feel for you?

9. As this is a lifestyle change and not a diet, write about what your life would look like and feel like in the maintenance phase. What would you do regularly? How would you feel? What would your daily meal plan look like? How would your relationship with food be similar or different? Describe this in detail.

10. How do you handle emotional issues in your life right now? How does it impact your eating behaviors?

11. How well do you handle life stressors? Describe your day-to-day life when you encounter stressful situations. How do you respond or react? How does it impact your eating behaviors?

Congratulations on RECOMMITING to your life, your health, and your long-term weight loss plan. I firmly believe you CAN and WILL release your weight regain. Go back through the prompts and guides throughout the book to help support you in creating your own strategy for success. Your success begins and ends with you. You can do ANYTHING you set your mind to!

REFERENCES

American Psychological Association. (2020). The impact of food advertising on childhood obesity. Retrieved from: https://www.apa.org/topics/kids-media/food

Atwood, M., David, L., & Cassin, S. (2017). Cognitive behavioral therapy for bariatric surgery patients. *Metabolism and Pathophysiology of Bariatric Surgery,* 595-603. doi:10.1016/b978-0-12-804011-9.00061-3

Axsom, D., & Cooper, J. (1985). Cognitive dissonance and psychotherapy: The role of effort justification in inducing weight loss. *Journal of Experimental Social Psychology, 21*(2), 149–160. Retrieved from: https://doi.org/10.1016/0022-1031(85)90012-5

Bardone-Cone, A. M. (2007). Self-oriented and socially prescribed perfectionism dimensions and their associations with disordered eating. *Behaviour Research and Therapy, 45*(8), 1977–1986. doi: 10.1016/j.brat.2006.10.004

Bond S., Phelan, S., Wolfe, L. G., Evans, R. K., Meador, J. G., Kellum, J. M., . . . Wing, R. R. (2009). Becoming physically active after bariatric surgery is associated with improved weight loss and health-related quality of life. *Obesity, 17*(1), 78-83. doi:10.1038/oby.2008.501

Bradley, L. E., Forman, E. M., Kerrigan, S. G., Goldstein, S. P., Butryn, M. L., Thomas, J. G., ... Sarwer, D. B. (2016). Project HELP: A Remotely

Delivered Behavioral Intervention for Weight Regain after Bariatric Surgery. *Obesity Surgery, 27*(3), 586–598. doi: 10.1007/s11695-016-2337-3

Burke, L. E., Wang, J., & Sevick, M. A. (2011). Self-Monitoring in Weight Loss: A Systematic Review of the Literature. *Journal of the American Dietetic Association, 111*(1), 92–102. doi: 10.1016/j.jada.2010.10.008

Butryn, M. L., Phelan, S., Hill, J. O., & Wing, R. R. (2007). Consistent Self-monitoring of Weight: A Key Component of Successful Weight Loss Maintenance. *Obesity, 15*(12), 3091–3096. doi: 10.1038/oby.2007.368

Cleveland Clinic. (2019, August 19). Study looks at ketogenic diet to treat PCOS and infertility. Consult QD. Retrieved from https://consultqd.clevelandclinic.org/study-looks-at-ketogenic-diet-to-treat-pcos-and-infertility/

Dweck, C. S. (2016). *Mindset: The new psychology of success*. New York: Ballantine Books.

Elrod, H. (2017). *The Miracle Morning: The not-so-obvious Secret Guaranteed to Transform Your Life Before 8AM*. Temecula, CA: Hal Elrod International, Inc.

Faden, J., Leonard, D., O'Reardon, J., & Hanson, R. (2013). Obesity as a defense mechanism. *International Journal of Surgery Case Reports, 4*(1), 127–129. doi: 10.1016/j.ijscr.2012.10.011

Freire, R. H., Borges, M. C., Alvarez-Leite, J. I., & Correia, M. I. (2012). Food quality, physical activity, and nutritional follow-up as determinant of weight regain after Roux-en-Y gastric bypass. *Nutrition, 28*(1), 53-58. doi:10.1016/j.nut.2011.01.011

Galletly, C., Moran, L., Noakes, M., Clifton, P., Tomlinson, L., & Norman, R. (2007). Psychological benefits of a high-protein, low-carbohydrate diet in obese women with polycystic ovary syndrome—A pilot study. *Appetite, 49*(3), 590–593. doi: 10.1016/j.appet.2007.03.222

Geraci, A., Brunt, A. R., & Hill, B. D. (2015). The pain of regain: Psychosocial impacts of weight regain among long-term bariatric patients. *Bariatric Surgical Practice and Patient Care, 10*(3), 110-118. doi:10.1089/bari.2015.0011

Handley, R. T., Bentley, R. E., Brown, T. L., & Annan, A. A. (2018). Successful treatment of obesity and insulin resistance via ketogenic diet status post Roux-en-Y. *BMJ Case Reports, 2018* doi:http://dx.doi.org.library.capella.edu/10.1136/bcr-2018-225643

Hartmann-Boyce, J., Boylan, A.-M., Jebb, S. A., & Aveyard, P. (2018). Experiences of Self-Monitoring in Self-Directed Weight Loss and Weight Loss Maintenance: Systematic Review of Qualitative Studies. *Qualitative Health Research, 29*(1), 124–134. doi: 10.1177/1049732318784815

Henderson, V. R., & Kelly, B. (2005). Food Advertising in the Age of Obesity: Content Analysis of Food Advertising on General Market and African American Television. *Journal of Nutrition Education and Behavior, 37*(4), 191–196. doi: 10.1016/s1499-4046(06)60245-5

Hoek, J., & Gendall, P. (2006). Advertising and Obesity: A Behavioral Perspective. *Journal of Health Communication, 11*(4), 409–423. doi: 10.1080/10810730600671888

Johnson, S. S., Paiva, A. L., Cummins, C. O., Johnson, J. L., Dyment, S. J., Wright, J. A., ... Sherman, K. (2008). Transtheoretical Model-based multiple behavior intervention for weight management: Effectiveness on a population basis. *Preventive Medicine, 46*(3), 238–246. doi: 10.1016/j.ypmed.2007.09.010

Jones, Cleator, J., & Yorke, J. (2016). Maintaining weight loss after bariatric surgery: When the spectator role is no longer enough. *Clinical Obesity, 6*(4), 249-258. doi:10.1111/cob.12152

Koball, A. M., Himes, S. M., Sim, L., Clark, M. M., Collazo-Clavell, M. L., Mundi, M., ... Grothe, K. B. (2015). Distress tolerance and psychological comorbidity in patients seeking bariatric surgery. *Obesity Surgery, 26*(7), 1559-1564. doi:10.1007/s11695-015-1926-x

Liebl, L., Barnason, S., & Hudson, D. B. (2016). Awakening: A qualitative study on maintaining weight loss after bariatric surgery. *Journal of Clinical Nursing, 25*(7-8), 951-961. doi:10.1111/jocn.13129

Lynch, A. (2016). When the honeymoon is over, the real work begins: gastric bypass patients' weight loss trajectories and dietary change experiences. *Social Science & Medicine, 151*, 241-249. doi:10.1016/j.socscimed.2015.12.024

Masood, A., Alsheddi, L., Alfayadh, L., Bukhari, B., Elawad, R., & Alfadda, A. A. (2019). Dietary and lifestyle factors serve as predictors of successful weight loss maintenance postbariatric surgery. *Journal of Obesity, 2019*, 1-6. doi:10.1155/2019/7295978

Mavropoulos, J., Yancy, W., Hepburn, J., & Westman, E. (2005). The effects of a low-carbohydrate ketogenic diet on polycystic ovary syndrome: A pilot study. *Nutrition & Metabolism, 2*(1), 35. doi:10.1186/1743-7075-2-35

Orciari, M. (2018, March 15). Fast food companies still target kids with marketing for unhealthy products. *YaleNews.* Retrieved from https://news.yale.edu/2013/11/04/fast-food-companies-still-target-kids-marketing-unhealthy-products

Prochaska, J. O., Johnson, S., & Lee, P. (1998). The transtheoretical model of behavior change. In S. A. Shumaker, E. B. Schron, J. K. Ockene, & W. L. McBee (Eds.), *The handbook of health behavior change* (p. 59–84). Springer Publishing Co.

Prochaska, J. O., & Marcus, B. H. (1994). The transtheoretical model: Applications to exercise. In R. K. Dishman (Ed.), *Advances in exercise adherence* (p. 161–180). Human Kinetics Publishers.

Prochaska, J. O., & Velicer, W. F. (1997). The Transtheoretical Model of Health Behavior Change. *American Journal of Health Promotion, 12*(1), 38–48. doi: 10.4278/0890-1171-12.1.38

Seligman, M. E. P. (2018). *Learned optimism.* London: Nicholas Brealey Publishing.

Shaefer, A. (2020, February 20). Maltodextrin: What Is It and Is It Safe? *Healthline.* Retrieved from https://www.healthline.com/health/food-nutrition/is-maltodextrin-bad-for-me#when-to-avoid-it

Silva, J. C. (2018, July 11). Maltodextrin: What it is, dangers, and substitutes. *Medical News Today.* Retrieved from https://www.medicalnewstoday.com/articles/322426#is-maltodextrin-safe

Silverman, Linda Kreger (1 January 1999). "Perfectionism." *Gifted Education International. 13*(3): 216–225. doi:10.1177/026142949901300303.

Spurlock, M., & Con (Film). (2004). *Supersize Me.* New York, N.Y.: Hart Sharp Video.

Steinig, J., Wagner, B., Shang, E., Dölemeyer, R., & Kersting, A. (2012). Sexual abuse in bariatric surgery candidates - impact on weight loss after surgery: a systematic review. *Obesity Reviews, 13*(10), 892–901. doi: 10.1111/j.1467-789x.2012.01003.x

Zimmerman, F. J., & Shimoga, S. V. (2014). The effects of food advertising and cognitive load on food choices. *BMC Public Health, 14*(1). doi: 10.1186/1471-2458-14-3

RESOURCES

Follow BARIATRIC MINDSET on social media:

Facebook: Bariatric Mindset

Instagram: Bariatric Mindset

Twitter: @barimindset

Pinterest: Bariatric Mindset

For additional support, Join our FREE Support Group on Facebook (Bariatric Mindset Mavens):

http://www.facebook.com/groups/bariatricmindset

Sign up for the FREE 4-week e-course video series delivered via email:

The Mindset Behind Your Macros

https://programs.bariatricmindset.com/macro

For additional Bariatric Nutrition Resources, check out My Bariatric Kitchen and join the FREE Facebook group for bariatric friendly recipes and up to date bariatric nutrition information:

www.ingramcontent.com/pod-product-compliance
Lightning Source LLC
Chambersburg PA
CBHW021409210526
45463CB00001B/280